DEVELOPMENTAL PROFILES
Birth to Six

DEVELOPMENTAL PROFILES
Birth to Six

K. Eileen Allen
Lynn R. Marotz

DELMAR PUBLISHERS INC.®

NOTICE TO THE READER

Cover photos by Catherine Hopkins

Delmar Staff
 Associate Editor: Jay Whitney
 Editing Manager: Barbara A. Christie
 Project Editor: Ruth East
 Production Coordinator: Lawrence Main
 Design Coordinator: Susan Mathews

For information, address Delmar Publishers Inc.
3 Columbia Circle, PO Box 15015
Albany, New York 12212–5015

Printed in the United States of America
Published simultaneously in Canada
by Nelson Canada,
A division of The Thomson Corporation

10 9 8

Library of Congress Cataloging in Publication Data
Allen, K. Eileen, 1918-
    Developmental profiles: birth to six / K. Eileen Allen, Lynn R. Marotz.
      p.   cm.
    Bibliography: p.
    Includes index.
    ISBN 0-8273-3355-2 (pbk.). ISBN 0-8273-3356-0 (instructor's guide)
    1. Child development. I. Marotz, Lynn R. II. Title.
RJ131.A496 1989   88-22912
155.4—dc19   CIP

Contents

Preface

Developmental Profiles: Birth to Six, is a handbook designed for

- child development and early childhood students and teachers-in-training;
- child-care providers in home care settings, day care centers, preschools and Head Start Programs, and nannies in the child's own home;
- allied health professionals from fields such as nursing, nutrition, audiology, medicine, social work and physical therapy;
- parents, who are always the most important contributors to a child's optimum development.

The handbook contains non-technical, basic knowledge about

- what to expect of young children at each succeeding stage of development;
- the ways in which all areas of development are intertwined and mutually supportive;
- the unique pathway that each child follows in a developmental process that is alike, yet different, among children of similar age;
- the concept of developmental sequences being the crucial factor in development, not the child's chronological age.

This handbook offers a number of special features:

- concise profiles of developmental areas at various age levels from birth to six;
- a section that briefly defines and describes the most commonly encountered terms and concepts in the child development literature;
- developmental alerts for each level, boxed separately for easy reference;
- descriptions of daily activities and routines typical of children at each level;
- where and how to get help if there is concern about a child's development;
- a comprehensive developmental checklist and growth charts to aid in the observation and screening process;
- sketches of the school-age child; the preschool child, toddlers, and infants;
- an annotated bibliography for back-up and additional readings on child development, screening and assessment, referral and information resources;
- appendices containing growth charts, reflex schedules, a sample health history form, and a number of other useful features.

Acknowledgements

We are indebted to our typists Adola J. Stocker, Judith Faye Scheff, and Margaret Williams whose understanding and skilled typing made it possible for us to meet some intense deadlines to complete this project.

To the editors at Delmar who have provided the encouragement and technical assistance to complete this project: Karen Lavroff-Hawkins for her foresight and help in getting this project off the ground; Jay Whitney, who inherited this project midstream; and Ruth East, our Project Editor.

To our families for their patience and understanding. And, to our reviewers, a special thanks for their contributions: Jeanne W. Arvidson, South Seattle Community College; Constance A. Spohn, SUNY-Cobleskill; and Jane Catalani, San Antonio College

The authors wish to thank NFER-NELSON for their cooperation with this adaptation of **FROM BIRTH TO FIVE YEARS** by Mary D. Sheridan.

K. Eileen Allen, Professor Emeritus
University of Kansas
Lynn R. Marotz
University of Kansas

Introduction

The purpose of this handbook is to provide a brief, yet comprehensive guide to the development of young children from birth to six years of age. The need for such a handbook is twofold. One is to ensure that effective learning experiences and developmentally appropriate guidance and discipline measures are used at home and in child-care and early education centers.

A second reason involves current research. There is strong evidence that early identification and **intervention** can limit the harmful effect of development problems or delays. Everyone who cares for and works with infants and young children should have on hand a readily available and concise set of developmental guidelines. These will assist in the observation and assessment of children to determine if each child is on a steady and healthy course of growth and development.

The style of this book is nontechnical. Research documentation, characteristic of child development textbooks, is intentionally omitted. Instead, there are uncluttered word pictures of the child in action at selected levels and across all areas of development. However, the developmental profiles and accompanying information are based upon current research as reflected in the brief annotated bibliography of child development texts (Appendix 5).

This handbook is intended to supplement a basic text on child development. The information provided is compatible with contemporary child development texts. At the same time, the handbook reflects the authors' synthesis of variations found from textbook to textbook. Occasionally, where there has been an almost equal split between the ways a given topic has been handled, the authors have made an arbitrary decision. Combining perceptual and cognitive developmental areas is a case in point. Some texts discuss the two areas separately, others combine them. Because of their many overlapping characteristics during the early years, perceptual and cognitive skills have been combined in this handbook.

Infancy and the early toddler months occupy what may appear to be a disproportionate number of pages. However, such an allocation is justified because of the amazing developmental changes that occur during the first 15 to 24 months. Never again will so many new and complex behaviors and skills be acquired in so short a time span. In addition, a major change has taken place in our society. More and more infants and very young children are spending greater numbers of hours each day in infant and child-

---

intervention—This is a term used to describe educational programs and treatments planned to improve children's ability to learn and function in society.

care centers. Therefore, it is essential that there be knowledgeable caregivers who understand infant and toddler development. The third justification has already been mentioned—the need for the earliest possible identification of potential problems and delays. New federal legislation (PL 99-457; see Chapter 8) provides funds for screening, assessment and intervention services for children from birth to six years. To take advantage of these services, those who care for infants and young children must learn to recognize very early signs of developmental problems. This handbook offers a concise set of developmental guidelines for that purpose.

The aim of this handbook is that it be of significant help to anyone involved with infants, toddlers, and preschool-age children. At no point should this handbook, *or any textbook*, be seen as an instrument for diagnosing a child's problems or delays. Instead, the purpose of these developmental guidelines is to provide quick and easily located information about the young child for parents, caregivers, teachers and health-care providers.

The importance of parent involvement is stressed throughout the book with emphasis placed on the frontline role of parents. It is they who are in a position to note possible problems and delays. By reporting their observations, parents can make significant contributions to the information pool on their child. Also emphasized is the importance of listening to parents. Teachers, practitioners and clinicians must respond to parents with genuine interest, finding ways to communicate with them effectively, and including parents as members of the developmental team.

The authors are well qualified to compile this handbook. Both have many years of first-hand experience in working with young children, parents, teachers and allied health-care professionals, as well as many years of teaching and research at the university level.

K. Eileen Allen began her career as a parent participant and then a lay teacher in a parent-cooperative preschool. She spent several years as head teacher in a classroom for four-year-olds in the Developmental Psychology Laboratory Preschool, University of Washington. Subsequently, because of her interest in children with developmental problems, she served as the Coordinator of Early Childhood Education and Research and as a member of an interdisciplinary child-study team at the Child Development and Mental Retardation Center, also at the University of Washington. In 1974, as a professor of Human Development and Family Life, she went to the University of Kansas where she continued to work with children, parents and teachers; taught graduate and undergraduate courses; and conducted research related to how young children learn. Professor Allen has published extensively. Her textbooks focus on childhood development and early education, children with developmental problems and special needs, and the workings of interdisciplinary child study teams.

Lynn R. Marotz brings her nursing background and clinical experience with young children to the field of early childhood where her prime interests lie in teacher training, early recognition of health impairments and the promotion of wellness among young children. She joined the faculty of the Edna A. Hill Child Development Laboratory at the University of Kansas in 1977 and currently serves as the Health and Safety Coordinator and Associate Director. She teaches a variety of courses and works closely with graduate and undergraduate students in the early-childhood teacher-training program. Her experience also includes extensive involvement with health screenings, communicating and working with parents and health professionals and the referral process. Lynn Marotz has made numerous presentations and authored publications on a variety of issues related to children's health, identification of illness and developmental conditions, environmental safety and nutrition.

Chapter 1

Principal Concepts in Child Development

To provide effective care and guidance for young children, it is essential to understand the principal concepts of child development. Each child's overall development and behavior can then be put into focus day by day. Such understanding also gives a long-range perspective on each child. This two-track approach is indispensible in helping all children grow and develop in ways best-suited to each of them as unique individuals.

The following key concepts have been selected because of their current importance and widespread use in the field of child development. Varied as these concepts are, it is necessary to understand and apply all of them in working effectively with infants and young children.

BASIC NEEDS

All children, whether normal, handicapped or **at-risk** for developmental problems, have a number of physical and psychological needs. These needs must be met if infants and children are to survive, thrive, and develop to their optimum potential. Many developmental psychologists view birth through five years of age as the most critical of any developmental period in the entire lifespan. Never again will the child be so totally dependent upon adults—parents, caregivers, teachers—to satisfy the basic needs of life and to provide opportunities for learning.

Although separated in the lists that follow, it must be understood at the outset that physical and psychological needs are interrelated and interdependent. Meeting a child's physical needs while neglecting psychological needs may lead to developmental problems. The opposite is also true—a child who is physically neglected frequently experiences trouble in learning and getting along with others.

Basic Physical Needs
- Shelter, protection from harm
- Food, nutritious and appropriate to age of child
- Warmth, adequate clothing

---

at-risk—This term is used to describe children who may be more likely to have developmental problems due to certain predisposing factors.

1

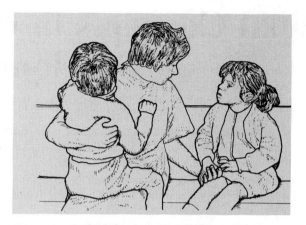

Children need affection.

- Preventive health and dental care, treatment of illnesses and physical problems, cleanliness
- Rest and activity, in balance.

Psychological Needs

- Affection and consistency—**nurturing** parents and caregivers who can be depended upon to be there.
- Security and trust—familiar surroundings with parents and caregivers who respond reliably and appropriately to the needs of the infant and child.
- Appropriate adult expectations as to what the child can and cannot do at each level of development.

---

nurturing—*Nurturing includes qualities of warmth, loving and caring.*

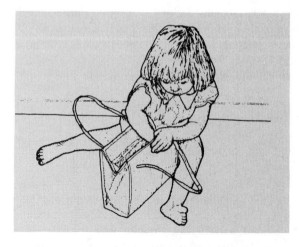

Children need freedom to explore.

The Need to Learn

- Freedom to explore and experiment with necessary limits clearly stated and consistently maintained.
- Access to developmentally appropriate experiences and play materials.
- An appropriate "match" between a child's skill levels and the materials and experiences available to the child: just enough newness to challenge, but not so much that the child feels overwhelmed, incapable or excessively frustrated.
- Errors, mistakes and failures treated as important steps in the learning process, never as reasons for condemning or ridiculing a child.
- Adults who demonstrate in everyday life the appropriate behaviors expected of the child, be it language, social interactions or ways of handling stress. *It must be remembered that parents, caregivers and teachers are major behavior models for young children.*

The Need for Respect

- A respectful and helpful environment in which the child's efforts are encouraged, approved and aided: "You picked up your crayons. Good job. Shall I put them on the shelf for you?"
- Acceptance of the child's efforts; respect for his or her accomplishments, small and large, errors as well as successes: "Look at that! You laced your shoes all by yourself." (No mention of the eyelet that was missed).
- Recognition that accomplishment, the "I can do" attitude is the major and most essential component of a child's **self-esteem:** "You're really getting good at cutting out cookies."

---

self-esteem—Feelings about oneself make up one's self-esteem.

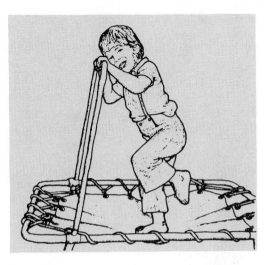

Children need respect for accomplishments.

- Sincere attention to what the child is doing well; helping the child learn to respect his or her own accomplishments through descriptive praise: "You got your shoes on the right feet all by yourself."
- Awareness of the tremendous amount of effort and concentration that goes into acquiring developmental skills; positive responses to each small step along the way as a child works toward mastery of a complex skill such as self-feeding with a spoon. "Right! Just a little applesauce on the spoon so it stays on."

NORMAL DEVELOPMENT

The concept of normal development is used in many different ways; therefore, it is difficult to define simply and specifically. In general, the term implies that a child is growing, changing and acquiring a broad range of skills according to some unobservable pattern or inner timetable. However, such a statement oversimplifies the concept of normal development. Several additional factors must be considered.

Development involves the following:

- An integrated process by which children change in orderly ways in terms of size, **neurological** structure and behavioral complexity.
- A cumulative or "building block" process; each new aspect of growth or development includes and builds upon earlier changes; each new behavioral or physical accomplishment is necessary to the next stage or next set of skills.
- A continuous process of give and take between the child and the environment; each changing the other in a variety of ways. (For example: The three-year-old drops a cup, breaks it and mother scolds the child. Both events, the broken cup

---

neurological—This term refers to the brain and nervous system.

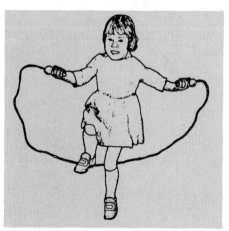

New skills are based on previously learned skills.

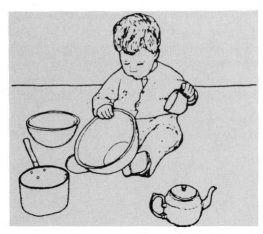

Development includes learning from experiences.

and mother's displeasure, are environmental changes that the child has created. From an experience like this the child may learn to hang on more firmly next time which constitutes a change in the child's behavior—fewer broken cups.)

A number of other key concepts also are closely related to the basic concept of normal development. These will be touched upon one by one.

Developmental Milestones

Developmental milestones are major markers or points of accomplishment in children's development. They are made up of important motor, social, cognitive and language skills. They show up in somewhat orderly steps and within fairly predictable age ranges. Essentially, milestone behaviors are those that most normally developing children are likely to display at approximately the same age. For example, almost every child begins to smile between four and ten weeks, speak a first word or two around twelve months. Both of these achievements (social smile, first words) are but two of a number of highly significant behavioral indications that a child's developmental progress is on track. The failure of one or more developmental milestones to appear within a reasonable range of time is a warning that a child may be developing a problem and should be observed closely.

Sequences of Development

A sequence or pattern of development consists of predictable steps along a developmental pathway common to the majority of children. Children must be able to roll over before they can sit and sit before they can stand. *It is the order in which children acquire these developmental skills, this is the critical consideration, not the child's age in months and years*. A sequence of development is an important indication that the child is moving steadily forward along a sound developmental **continuum**. In language

continuum—A continuous pathway is a continuum.

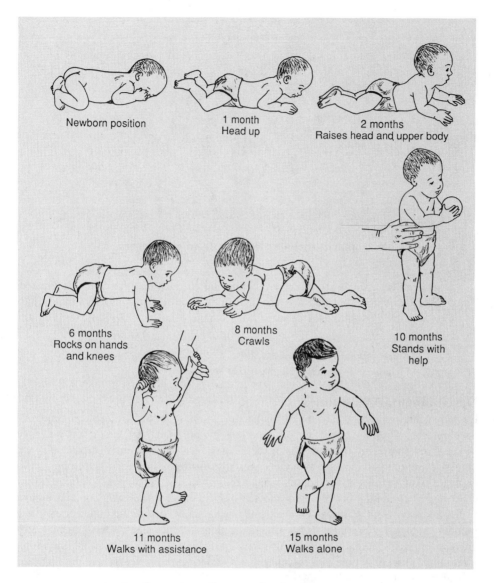

Sequences of motor development

development, for example, it does not matter how many words a child speaks by two years of age. What is important is that the child has progressed from cooing to babbling to "jabbering" (inflected jargon), to syllable production. The two-year-old who has progressed through those stages will almost surely produce words and sentences within a reasonable period of time.

It should be emphasized, however, that developmental progress is rarely smooth and even. Irregularities, such as periods of **stammering** or a **food jag**, characterize development. Regression, that is taking a step or two backward now and again, is perfectly normal and also to be expected. It is not unusual for a child who has been toilet trained to begin to have "accidents" when starting preschool or day care.

Age-Level Expectancies or Norms

Age-level expectancies can be thought of as chronological or age-related levels of development. Investigators like Arnold Gesell, Nancy Bailey and William Frankenburg carried out systematic observations on vast numbers of infants and children of various ages. Analyses of their findings represent the average or "normal" age at which many specifically described developmental skills are acquired by most children in a given culture. This average age is often called the norm; thus, a child's development may be described as at the norm, above the norm or below the norm. For example, a child who walks at 8 1/2 months is well below the norm of 12 to 15 months, while a child who does not walk until 20 months is well above the norm.

One point must be stressed: age-level expectancies *always represent a range and never an exact point in time* when specific skills will be achieved. Profiles of age expectancies for specific skills should always be interpreted as approximate mid-points on a range of months (as in the example walking, from 8 to 20 months with the midpoint at 14 months.) Once again, a reminder: it is *sequence* and *not age* that is the important factor in evaluating a child's progress.

Range of Normalcy

In real life, there is probably no child who is truly normal in every way. The range of skills and the age at which skills are acquired show great variation. This is true even among children who are described as being typical or as developing normally. Relevant again is the example of walking, one infant starting at 8 ½ months and another not until 20 months. Both are within the normal range, though many months apart on either side of the norm. No two children grow and develop at exactly the same rate, nor do they perform in exactly the same way. There are a half-dozen perfectly normal ways of creeping and crawling. Most children, however, use what is referred to as contralateral locomotion, an opposite knee-hand method of getting about, prior to walking. Also, some normally walking two-year-olds never crawled. Thus, normalcy encompasses great variation and a wide range of differences among individual children.

Developmental Transitions and Consolidations

Development can be thought of as a series of phases. Spurts of rapid growth and development are often followed by periods of disorganization or disequilibrium. Then the child seems to recover and again go into a time of reorganization. It is not at all

---

stammering—To stutter or speak in an interrupted pattern is stammering.

food jag—A period when only a certain food is preferred or accepted is called a food jag.

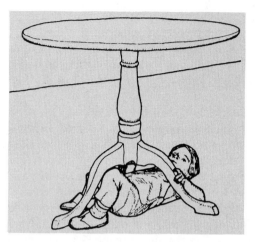

**Behavior problems are not uncommon
during transitions and consolidations.**

uncommon for children to demonstrate behavior problems or even regression during any one of these periods. The reasons vary. Perhaps the new baby has become an active and engaging older infant who is now the center of family attention. Three-year-old brother may revert to babyish ways about the same time. He begins to have tantrums over minor frustrations. He loses, for the time being, his hard-won bladder control. Usually, these transition periods are short-lived. The three-year-old, for example, almost always will learn more age-appropriate ways of getting attention.

Interrelatedness of Developmental Areas

As noted in the beginning, discussions about development usually divide it into several major components or areas. These areas carry labels such as physical, motor, perceptual, cognitive, personal-social and language. However, no one area ever develops independently of other developmental areas. Every skill, whether simple or complex, is a mixture. Social skills are a good example. Why are some young children said to have good social skills? Often the answer is because they play well with other children and are sought after as playmates. But to be a preferred playmate, a child must have many skills. A four-year-old, for example, must be able to do all of the following:

- Run, jump, climb and build with blocks (good motor skills)
- Ask for, explain and describe what is going on (good language skills)
- Recognize likenesses and differences among play materials and so select the right materials in a joint building project (good perceptual skills)
- Problem solve, conceptualize and plan ahead in cooperative play ventures (good cognitive skills).

Every developmental area is equally well-represented in the above example, even though social development was the area under consideration.

Heredity and Environment (sometimes called the nature/nurture controversy)

Each child has a unique **genetic** makeup. Genetic makeup influences a child's temperament or disposition, energy level, and rate of physical and intellectual development. However, no aspect of a child's makeup, except perhaps eye color, hair color, shape of nose and certain other physical characteristics, can be attributed exclusively to either heredity (internal influences) or to environment (external influences). From the moment of conception, both factors continuously interact and contribute to the child's overall pattern of growth and development.

Maturation

Maturation implies changes in the infant or child that are biological rather than learned. In other words, maturation is the appearance of new skills or behaviors common to all developing human beings. Sitting, walking and talking are examples of maturation. As noted earlier, these skills do not come about independently of the environment. Learning to walk, for example, involves muscle strength and coordination (influenced by adequate nutrition). Learning to walk also requires an environment that encourages practice, not only of walking as it emerges, but also of the behaviors and skills that preceded walking, such as rolling over, sitting and crawling.

Individual Differences

A number of factors contribute to making each child unique, special, different from every other child. Genetic inheritance and environment have been discussed. Several additional factors will be touched upon next.

Temperament. Temperament is the term used to describe an individual's patterns of behaviors or responses to everyday happenings. Infants and young children are different from each other in their activity level, alertness, irritability, soothability, restlessness and cuddliness. Such qualities often lead to labels—the "good" child, the "difficult" child, the "aggressive" child. These characteristics (and labels) seem to have a definite effect on the ways that family, caregivers and teachers respond to the child. This in turn, reinforces the child's self perceptions. For example, a hostile child is often treated with hostility by others. This treatment, in turn, tends to justify to the child his or her hostile behaviors.

Sex Roles. Early in life, young children learn the sex roles that are considered appropriate by their culture. Each boy and girl develops a set of behaviors, attitudes and commitments that are defined for them, directly or indirectly, as being acceptable male or female behaviors. In addition, each child plays out sex roles according to everyday experiences. In other words, each child's sex role development will be influenced by playmates and play opportunities, toys, type and amount of television and especially by adult models (parents, neighbors, teachers).

---

genetic—This term refers to inherited biological qualities.

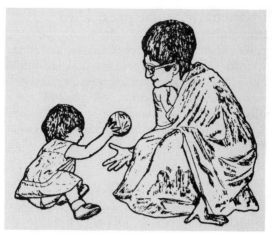

**Cultural and socio-economic factors
influence development before birth.**

Culture and Socio-economic Factors. Long before birth, cultural and economic factors begin to influence the child's uniqueness. These influences include the following:

- General health and nutrition of the mother
- The mother's understanding of her obligations and responsibilities to her unborn child
- Availability of pre- and post-natal medical care
- Ethnic and religious beliefs and practices.

Factors such as these contribute to each child being unlike any other child. For example, the child born to a single, fifteen-year-old mother living in poverty will be very different from a child born and raised in a two-parent, middle-class, professional family.

Transactional Patterns of Development

From birth, the child begins to influence the behavior of parents and caregivers. In turn, parents and caregivers are influencing the child. Thus, development is a reciprocal, or give-and-take process, between a child and significant adults. In other words, parents, caregivers, teachers and child are continuously interacting in ways that influence each other's behaviors and development. For example, a calm, cuddly baby expresses its needs in a clear and predictable fashion. This infant begins life with personal-social experiences that are quite different from those of a tense, colicky infant whose sleeping and eating patterns are highly irregular and, therefore, stressful to parents. The transactional process between infants and parents will be quite different in each of these instances and so will the developmental outcome.

Contingent Stimulation

A concept appearing in several recent child-development texts is contingent stimulation. The term refers to the specific ways in which parents and caregivers respond to a child's efforts to get attention. Children thrive when adults respond promptly and positively, at least a fair share of the time, to appropriate things a child says and does. Developmental research supports that statement. Children develop healthier self-concepts, as well as earlier and better language, congnitive and social skills if raised with responsive adults. Contingent stimulation, therefore, must not be overlooked as a major factor in facilitating a child's progress in all areas of development.

ATYPICAL DEVELOPMENT

The term atypical is used to describe children with developmental problems—children whose development appears to be incomplete or inconsistent with normal patterns and sequences. These children are often said to be either delayed or different in their development, even handicapped. The child with developmental delays can be described as one who is performing in one or more areas of development like a much younger, normal child. The child who is still babbling with no recognizable words at age three is an example of delayed development. This condition need not be handicapping unless the child never develops **functional language**. Developmental deviation refers to an aspect of development that is different from what is ever seen in a normally developing child. The child born with six toes or with a profound hearing loss has a developmental deviation. The six-toed child is not likely to be considered handicapped while the deaf child has a serious and perhaps life-long handicap.

In conclusion, this brief discussion of significant principles and concepts related to child development is intended to refresh, enhance and update the readers' understanding of the developing child. The developmental profiles that follow will have greater meaning and value when used in the context of these basic principles and concepts.

---

functional language—*Language that yields the desired outcome is functional language.*

REVIEW QUESTIONS

1. List three psychological needs of the developing child.
   a.

   b.

   c.

2. List three terms related to normal developmental progression.
   a.

   b.

   c.

3. List three ways in which an adult can show respect for a young child's accomplishments.
   a.

   b.

   c.

TRUE OR FALSE

1. All that a child needs to develop fully is adequate food, warm housing, adequate clothing and good medical attention.

2. Errors, mistakes and failures displayed by a young child provide opportunities for learning.

3. Each new accomplishment in a young child's development is built upon earlier skills and experiences.

4. Environment has very little effect on a child's long-term development.

5. Maturation is biologically based (for the most part) and includes such things as learning to sit up, crawl and walk.

6. The child with developmental delays is handicapped throughout life.

MULTIPLE CHOICE. Select one or more correct answers from the lists below.

1. All areas of development are
   a. interrelated.
   b. interdependent.
   c. influenced by environment.

2. Development is
   a. cumulative, a building-block process.
   b. independent of neurological structure.
   c. physically and psychologically interactive.

3. Most normally developing children
   a. begin to smile between four and ten weeks.
   b. walk no later then one year.
   c. should be talking in sentences by two years of age.

4. Development can be thought of as a series of phases that
   a. all children go through at the same age.
   b. show no regression; that is, the child always goes forward, never backwards.
   c. influenced by economic and cultural factors.

5. Children develop healthier self concepts when adults provide
   a. contingent stimulation.
   b. frequent criticism and correction of errors the child makes.
   c. ample praise, especially descriptive praise.

Chapter 2

Growth and Development: What Is It?

GROWTH AND DEVELOPMENT

Growth and development are terms that often are used interchangeably. Yet, they are not identical concepts. Each refers to distinct aspects of the life process.

Growth refers to specific changes and increases in the child's actual size. Additional numbers of cells, as well as an increase in the size of existing cells, account for the observable increases in a child's height, weight, head circumference, shoe size, length of arms and legs and body shape. All growth changes lend themselves to direct and fairly reliable measurement.

The growth process is continuous throughout a child's life span. However, the rate of growth varies considerably according to age. For example, growth occurs rapidly during infancy and adolescence. In contrast, growth is slower and less dramatic in the preschool-aged child and in the adult. Yet even when the child reaches adulthood, the body continues to repair and replace its cells.

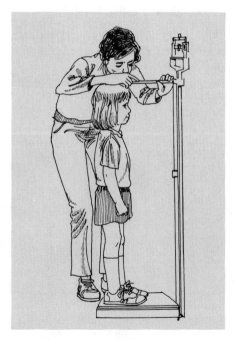

Growth is an increase in size.

Development refers to an increase in complexity, a change from relatively simple to more complicated. Development is a term that refers to an orderly progression along a continuous pathway on which the child acquires more refined knowledge, behaviors and skills. The sequence is basically the same for all children. However, the rate of development, as noted in Chapter 1, varies from child to child.

A child's rate and level of development are closely related to physiological maturity, especially of the nervous and muscular systems. Also, development is influenced by biological makeup (heredity) and environmental factors that are unique to each individual. Together, these factors account for the range of variations that can be seen in individual children's developmental achievements.

Normal growth and development is a term used to indicate **acquisition** of certain skills and behaviors according to a predictable rate and sequence. As noted in Chapter 1, the range of what is considered normal is broad. It includes mild variations or simple irregularities: the three-year-old who lisps, the twelve-month-old who learns to walk without having crawled.

At-risk is a phrase used to describe infants and young children who have a high probability of developing problems: newborns who were premature and of low-birth-weight; infants whose mothers had poor nutrition; children of teen-age parents. Early identification and intervention are of crucial importance with infants and children at-risk for developmental problems.

The term *atypical* is used to describe a child's growth or development that is incomplete or inconsistent with the normal sequence. Abnormal development in one area may or may not interfere with the development and mastery of skills in other areas. There are many reasons for atypical development including genetic abnormalities, poor nutrition, illness, injury, lack of opportunities to learn and impoverished environments.

DEVELOPMENTAL AREAS

To describe and assess accurately children's developmental progress, it is necessary to have a framework within which to work. For discussion purposes in this and other basic child-development textbooks, six major developmental areas have been identified: growth and physical development; motor; perceptual; cognitive; speech and language; personal-social. Each area includes many kinds of skills and behaviors, which will be discussed in the developmental profiles that follow. Although these developmental areas, as noted earlier, are separated for the purpose of discussion, they cannot be separated from one another in reality. Each is integrally related to, and interdependent with, each of the others.

***acquisition**—This means the process of learning or achieving specific objectives has been accomplished.*

Developmental profiles or "word pictures" are useful for assessing the current and on-going status of childrens' skills and behavior. It is important to keep in mind that the rate of development is uneven and occasionally unpredictable across areas, especially during the first two years of a child's life. For example, the language and social skills of infants and toddlers are less well-developed than their ability to move about. Also, children's individual achievements may vary across all developmental areas: A child may walk late but talk early. Again, an important reminder: Development in any of the areas is dependent on children having appropriate stimulation and opportunities to learn.

Physical development and growth are the major tasks of early infancy and childhood. Governed by heredity and greatly influenced by environmental conditions, physical development and growth is a highly individualized process. It is responsible for changes in body shape and proportions as well as for increase in overall body size. Growth, and especially growth of the brain, occurs more rapidly during the first year than at any other time. Growth is intricately related to progress in other developmental areas, too. It results in increased muscle strength for movement, depth perception in reaching for objects, and improved muscular control for bladder training. The state of a child's physical development serves as a reliable index of general health and well-being. It also has a direct influence on determining whether children are likely to achieve their potential in each of the other developmental areas, including intellectual achievement.

Motor development refers to a child's ability to move about and control various body parts. Refinements in motor development depend on maturation of the brain, input from the sensory system, increased bulk and number of muscle fibers and a healthy nervous system.

Motor abilities during early infancy are purely **reflexive**; most of them gradually disappear as the child develops **voluntary** control. If these earliest reflexes do not

---

reflexive—*Acts or movements resulting from impulses of the nervous system that cannot be controlled by the individual are reflexive.*

voluntary—*Movements that can be willed and purposively controlled and initiated by the individual are voluntary.*

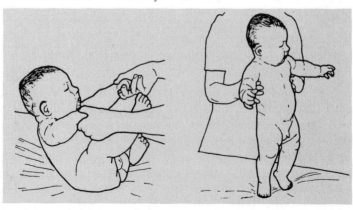

Cephalo-caudal development proceeds from head to toe.

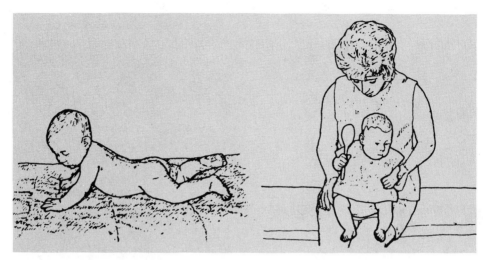

Proximo-distal development proceeds from trunk to arms and legs.

phase out at appropriate times in the developmental sequence, it may be an indication of neurological problems (see Appendix). In such cases, medical evaluation should be sought.

Three principles of maturation appear to govern motor development:

1. *Cephalo-caudal*: muscular development that proceeds from head to toe. The infant first learns to control muscles that support the head and neck, later those that allow reaching for objects, and then muscles for walking.
2. *Proximo-distal*: muscular development that begins with improved control of muscles closest to the central portion of the body, gradually moving outward and away from the midpoint to the extremities (arms and legs). Control of the head and neck is achieved before the child can pick up an object with thumb and forefinger (pincer grasp or finger-thumb opposition).
3. *Refinement*: muscular development that progresses from general or **gross motor** control used in sitting up or walking, to specific fine motor control, such as feeding self with a spoon.

Perceptual development refers to the increasingly complex use the child makes of information received through the senses: sight, hearing, touch, smell, taste and body position. In one sense, perception is concerned with how to use any one or any combinations of the senses. Perception also relates to learning to select specific aspects of the environment on which to focus. In other words, which details of a situation are important? Which differences should be noted? Which should be ignored? Even these simple questions point up how difficult, if not impossible, it is to separate perceptual

---

***gross motor**—Gross motor skills involve large muscle movements: walking, running, reaching.*

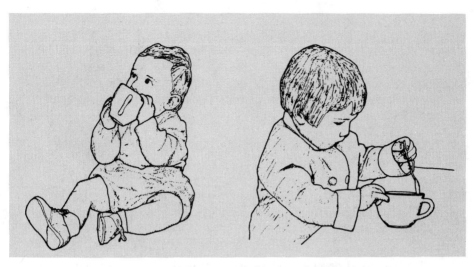

Refinement means an improved skill.

processes from cognitive processes. Separating perceptual from cognitive processes is a problem that was encountered again and again in preparing the profiles that follow. It led to the decision to combine perception and cognition at every age level throughout infancy and early childhood.

Three important aspects of perceptual development need to be mentioned:.

1. *Multi-modality*: Information from the environment is generally received through more than one sense organ at a time; when listening to a speaker, we use sight (watching facial expressions and mouth movements) and sound (listening to the words).

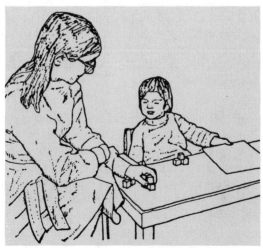

Multi-modality means the child uses information gathered by many senses.

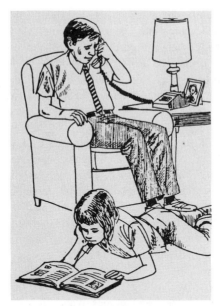

Habituation

2. *Habituation*: This is the ability to ignore whatever is not relevant or most important to the immediate situation; the child who is unaware of a dog barking in the background and focuses instead on the story that is being read.
3. *Sensory integration*: The child translates **sensory information** into intelligent behavior; the five-year-old sees and hears a car coming and waits on the curb for it to pass.

---

sensory information—*Sensory information is information received through the senses: eyes, ears, nose, mouth, touch.*

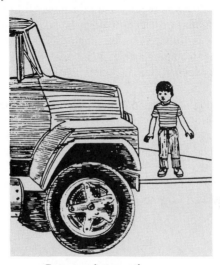

Sensory integration

The entire perceptual system is in place at the time of birth. Through experience, learning and maturation, it develops into a smoothly coordinated system for processing complex information (sorting shapes according to size and color) and making fine discriminations (telling the difference among initial sounds in rhyming words such as rake, cake, lake). The sensory system also enables an individual to respond appropriately to all kinds of messages and signals: smiling in response to a smile; keeping quiet in response to a frown.

Cognitive development has to do with the expansion of a child's intellect or mental abilities. Cognition is finding, processing, and organizing information and then using the information appropriately. The cognitive process includes such mental activities as discovering, interpreting, sorting and classifying and remembering information. In older children it means evaluating ideas, making judgements, solving problems, understanding rules and concepts, thinking ahead and visualizing possibilities or consequences. Cognitive development is an ongoing process of interaction between the child and objects or events in the environment.

Cognitive development begins with the reflexive behaviors that permit survival and primitive learning in the newborn. Next comes what Piaget has labelled the stage of sensory-motor activity. This stage lasts until approximately age two. The sensory-motor period is followed by a time of preoperational activity (another Piagetian term) that allows young children to internally process information coming in through their senses. Again it must be stressed that it is difficult, if not impossible, to discuss cognition as a separate developmental area, especially in the earliest years. Always there is considerable overlap with both perceptual development and motor involvement. As the child matures, a further complication comes about—the overlap with language development.

Language Development Language is often defined as a system of symbols, both spoken and written. It is a system that allows humans to communicate with one another. Normal *language development* is regular and sequential. It depends upon maturation as well as learning opportunities. The first year of life is called the prelinguistic or prelanguage phase. This is followed by the linguistic or language stage where speech becomes the major way of communicating. Words and grammatical rules are learned as children gain skill in conveying their thoughts and ideas through language.

In terms of speech and language development, children seem to understand concepts and relationships long before they have the words to describe them. In other words, receptive language (understanding what is said) precedes expressive language (the ability to use words to describe and explain). It appears obvious that speech and language development depends on, and is related to the child's general cognitive development. However, language development also depends on the type of language the child hears as well as genetic influences and maturation of the neuromuscular system.

Personal and social development is a broad area that concerns how children feel about themselves and their relationships with others. It refers to children's individual behaviors and responses to play and work activities, attachments to parents and caregivers and relationships with brothers, sisters and friends. Sex roles, independence, morality, trust, accepting rules and laws—these, too, are basic aspects of personal and social development. The family and its cultural values and differences are influential factors in shaping a child's social development and determining much of a child's basic personality.

In describing personal and social development, it must be remembered once again that children develop at different rates. Individual differences in genetic endowment, cultural background, health status and a host of other environmental factors contribute to these differences. Therefore, no two children can ever be exactly alike, not in social development or in any other area of development.

AGE DIVISIONS

The age divisions used throughout this book are based to some degree on those that Piaget and many child developmentalists use when describing significant changes within developmental areas:

Infant—	0–28 days (neonate, newborn)
	1–4 months
	4–8 months
	8–12 months
Toddler—	12–18 months
	1½–2 years
Preschool—	3rd, 4th, and 5th years

These age divisions are consistent with many of the current child development textbooks. Nevertheless, they are to be used with extreme caution and great flexibility when dealing with real children. They are based on the averaged achievements, abilities and behaviors of many children at various points in development. As has been stated again and again, there is great variation from one child to another, and IT IS SEQUENCE, NOT AGE, that is the major index to development.

In conclusion, this chapter provides a review of common terms and definitions used to describe the major developmental areas. These terms are the foundation upon which the profiles have been developed. It is important that everyone working with young children understand the concepts and their many variations in order to use the profiles effectively.

REVIEW QUESTIONS

1. List three factors thar are related to a child's rate of development.
   a.

   b.

   c.

2. List three factors that may lead to atypical or abnormal development.
   a.

   b.

   c.

3. List three sources of perceptual information.
   a.

   b.

   c.

TRUE OR FALSE

1. The terms growth and development can be used interchangeably because they mean exactly the same thing.

2. The rate at which a child develops is identical to all other children of the same age and sex.

3. Premature infants are often at-risk for developmental problems.

4. Malnutrition during the mother's pregnancy can have a damaging effect on the child's development after it is born.

5. Growth of the brain occurs more rapidly during the infant's first year than at any other time during life.

6. Perceptual development depends upon what the infant sees, hears, smells, tastes and touches.

7. The entire perceptual system is in place at the time of birth.

8. Receptive language develops after expressive language.

MULTIPLE CHOICE Select one or more correct answers from the lists below.

1. Development is
   a. a change from simple to complex skills.
   b. a sequential process that is basically the same for all children.
   c. variable in terms of rate—that, is some children may walk earlier than others but talk later and still be considered normal.

2. Motor development during early infancy
   a. is almost entirely reflexive.
   b. is not associated with cognitive development.
   c. can he speeded up with direct teaching and practice.

3. Which of following terms are associated with motor development?
   a. sensory integration
   b. proximo-distal
   c. cephalo-caudal

4. Which of the following terms are important to perceptual development?
   a. sensory integration
   b. racial integration
   c. school integration

5. Personal and social development are influenced by
   a. heredity.
   b. general health.
   c. culture and race.

6. Growth is
   a. measurable.
   b. faster during the preschool years than during infancy.
   c. continuous, in one form or an other throughout most of life.

Chapter 3

The Infant

NEWBORN BIRTH to 28 DAYS

The newborn infant is truly amazing. Within moments of birth it begins to adapt to an outside world that is radically different from the one experienced **in utero**. Furthermore, all body systems are in place and ready to function at the time of birth. The newborn's body is able immediately to assume responsibility for breathing, eating, eliminating, and regulating its body temperature; however, these systems are still immature and the newborn is completely dependent on parents and caregivers for survival.

Motor development (movement) is both reflexive and protective. There is no voluntary control of the body during the early weeks. Although newborn babies sleep most of the time, they are not passive. They are sensitive to their environment and have unique methods of responding to it. Crying is their primary method of communicating and expressing emotions. Certain perceptual and cognitive abilities are present, but they are almost impossible to distinguish from one another at this stage.

DEVELOPMENTAL PROFILES AND GROWTH PATTERNS

Growth and Physical Characteristics

The newborn's physical characteristics during the first few days of life are different from those of a slightly older infant. The skin is wrinkled. Within the first few days it will dry out and possibly peel in some areas. Skin color of all babies is relatively light but will gradually darken to a shade characteristic of their racial background. The head may appear to have an unusual shape as a result of the birth process, but it will return to a normal shape within the first week. Hair color and the amount of hair varies with the individual baby.

- Average weight range at birth is 6.5 to 9 pounds (2.9–4.0 kg); females weigh approximately 7 pounds (3.15 kg) and males approximately 7 pounds, 5 ounces (3.3 kg).
- Five to seven percent of birth weight is lost in the immediate days following birth.
- Average length at birth ranges from 18 to 21 inches (45.7–53.3 cm).
- An average of 5 to 6 ounces per week is gained during the first month.

---

in utero—*This term refers to growth of the fetus (developing baby) in the mother's uterus before birth.*

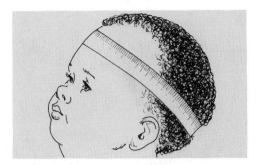

Head circumference

- Respiration (breathing) rate is approximately 30 to 50 breaths per minute.
- Chest appears small and cylindrical; it is nearly the same size as the head.
- Normal body temperature ranges from 96F. to 99F.(35.6–37.2 C).
- Regulation of body temperatures is difficult during the first few weeks due to immature body systems and the thin layer of fat beneath the skin.
- Heart rate (pulse) ranges from 120 to 150 beats per minute and may be irregular at times.
- Skin is sensitive, especially on the hands and mouth.
- Head is large in relation to body; accounts for nearly one-fourth of the total body length.
- Head circumference averages 12.5 to 14.5 inches (31.7–36.8 cm) at birth.
- "Soft" spots (**fontanels**) are located on the top (anterior) and back (posterior) of the head.
- Breathing is **abdominal** (rather than from the chest) and often irregular in rhythm and rate.
- Tongue appears large in proportion to the mouth.
- Visual acuity thought to be approximately 20/100–20/200.
- Crying is without tears.

---

fontanels—These small openings in the infant's skull bones are covered with a soft tissue and eventually grow closed; sometimes called "soft spots."
abdominal—This refers to the lower abdomen or "stomach" region.

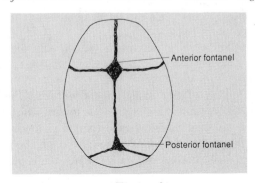

Fontanels

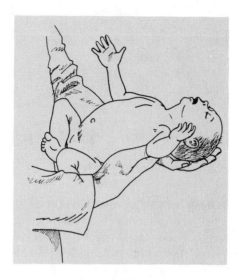

Moro reflex

Motor Development

The newborn's motor skills are purely reflexive movements such as those listed below. These movements are designed primarily for protection and survival. During the first month, the infant begins to gain some control over several of these early reflexes.

- Engages in motor activity that is primarily reflexive:
    —Swallowing, sucking, gagging, coughing, yawning, blinking and elimination reflexes are present at birth.
    —Rooting reflex is triggered by gently touching sensitive skin around the cheek and mouth; the infant turns toward the cheek being stroked.
    —Startle reflex is set off by sudden, loud noises; both arms are thrown open and away from the body, then quickly returned.
    —Moro reflex is brought about by quickly lowering the infant's position downward (as if dropping); arms are thrown open and quickly brought back together over the chest.
    —Grasping reflex occurs when the infant tightly curls its fingers around an object placed in its hand.
    —Stepping reflex involves the infant moving the feet up and down in walking-like movements when held upright with feet touching a firm surface.
    —Tonic neck reflex (TNR) occurs when the infant, in supine (face up) position, extends arm and leg on the side toward which the head is turned; the opposite arm and leg are flexed (pulled in toward the body); this is sometimes called the "fencing position."
    —Plantar reflex is the curling of toes when pressure is placed against the ball of foot.
- Maintains "fetal" position (back flexed or rounded, extremities held close to the body, knees drawn up) especially when asleep.

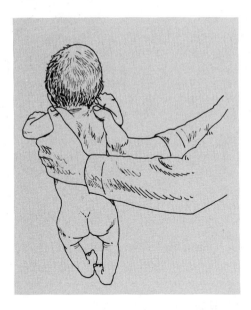

Stepping reflex

- Holds hands in a fist; does not reach for objects.
- When held in a prone (face down) position, baby's head falls lower than the horizontal line of the body with hips flexed and arms and legs hanging downward.
- Has good muscle tone in the upper body when held up and supported under the arms.
- Turns head from side to side when placed in a prone (face down) position.
- **Pupils** dilate (enlarge) and constrict (become smaller).

pupils—*Pupils are the small, dark, central portion of the eye.*

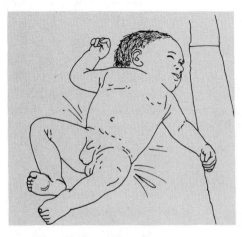

Tonic neck reflex

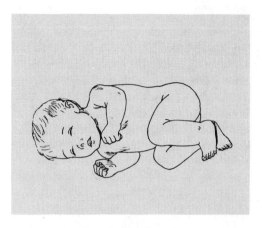

Sleeping in fetal position

Perceptual-Cognitive Development

The perceptual-cognitive skills of the newborn are designed to capture and hold the attention of parents and caregivers and to gain some sense of the environment. Hearing is the best developed of the perceptual skills. Newborns can hear and respond to differences among certain sounds and are especially responsive to mother's voice. Sounds and movements such as crooning, rocking and jiggling seem to be soothing. Newborns also respond to being touched over most of the body, with mouth and hands being the most sensitive. Vision is present, although limited. The newborn can focus both eyes, see objects up close and follow slowly moving objects. Newborns are also capable of learning. From the earliest days of life, they are taking in information through all of their senses. In other words they are gathering information from what they see, hear, touch, taste and smell. Purely reflexive behaviors are the major characteristic of the newborn's cognitive efforts. These take the form of sucking, startle responses, grimacing, flailing of arms and legs and eye movements. As noted earlier, these responses overlap with perceptual responses.

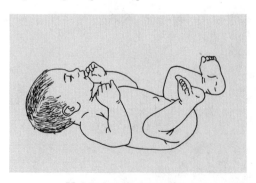

Holds hands in a fist

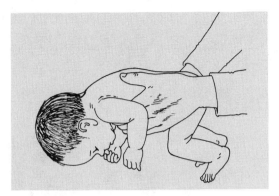

Prone suspension

- Eyes are extremely sensitive to light.
- Sees outlines and shapes; unable to focus on distant objects.
- Eyes do not always work together and may appear crossed at times.
- Makes somewhat coordinated eye and head movements to track (follow) objects that are out of direct line of vision.
- Gives a partial irregular eye blink to a fast-approaching object.
- Follows a slowly moving object through a complete arc of 180 degrees.
- Follows objects moved vertically (up and down) if object is close to infant's face.
- Shows defensive or self-protective reactions such as irregular eyeblinks to fast-approaching objects.
- Continues looking about even in the dark.
- Begins to study own hand when lying in tonic neck reflex (TNR) position.
- Hearing is present at birth and is more acute than vision. Infants hear as well as adults, except for quiet sounds.
- Prefers to listen to mother's voice than to a stranger's.
- Often synchronizes body movements to speech patterns of a parent or caregiver.
- Distinguishes some tastes; shows preference for sweet liquids.
- Sense of smell present at birth; will turn away from strong, unpleasant odors.

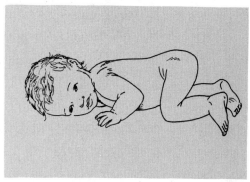

Studies own hand

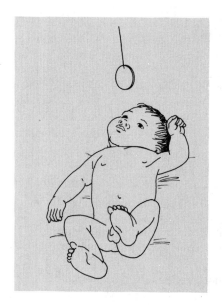

Follows vertically moving objects

Speech and Language

The beginnings of speech and language development can be identified in several of the newborn's reflexes. These include the bite-release action that occurs when the infant's gums are rubbed, the rooting reflex, and the sucking reflex. In addition, the new baby communicates directly and indirectly in a number of other ways.

- Reacts to loud auditory stimuli (noise) by blinking, moving a body part, stopping a movement, shifting eyes about, or making a startle response.
- Shows a preference for certain sounds, such as music and human voices by calming down or quieting.
- Turns head in response to voice on either side.
- Occasionally makes sounds other than crying.

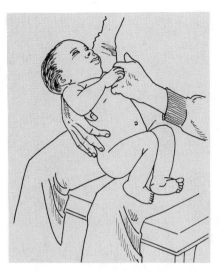

Stops crying when held

Personal-Social Development

Newborns are quite skilled at interacting socially. They are able to indicate needs and distress and to respond to parent's or caregiver's reactions to these behaviors. The very young infant thrives on feelings of security and soon displays a sense of attachment to primary caregivers.

- Experiences a short period of alertness immediately following birth.
- Sleeps 17 to 19 hours per day; gradually is awake and active for longer times.
- Likes to be held close and cuddled when awake.
- Shows qualities of individuality; each infant varies in ways of responding or not responding to the same situations.
- Begins to establish emotional attachment or "**bonding**" relationship with parents and caregivers.
- Expresses needs and emotions with unique cries and patterns of vocalizations that can be distinguished from one another.
- Stops crying when picked up and held.
- Begins to develop a sense of security or feeling of trust with parents and caregivers; responses to different individuals vary. For example, the infant may become tense with a caregiver who is uncomfortable with infant.

---

bonding—*The establishment of a close, loving relationship between an infant and adult, usually the mother and father, is called bonding.*

DAILY ROUTINES—BIRTH TO 28 DAYS

Eating

- Takes 6 to 8 feedings per 24 hours at the beginning of this period; later the number will be reduced to 5 or 6.
- Drinks 6 to 8 ounces of breast milk or formula per feeding.
- Takes from 25 to 30 minutes to complete a feeding.
- Expresses the need for food by crying.

Bathing, Dressing, Toileting Needs

- Signals the need for a diaper change by crying (if crying does not stop when diaper has been changed another reason for crying should be sought).
- Enjoys bath; keeps eyes open and gives other indications of pleasure when placed in warm water.
- Expresses displeasure when clothes are pulled over head (best to avoid over-the-head-clothes if possible).
- Enjoys being wrapped firmly (swaddled) in a blanket; swaddling seems to foster feelings of warmth and security.
- Has one to 4 bowel movements per day.

Sleeping

- Has 4 to 6 sleep periods per 24 hours; one of these is 5 to 7 hours in length.
- Falls asleep toward the end of nursing.
- Cries before falling asleep (usually stops if held and rocked briefly).

Play and Social Activities

- Enjoys light and brightness; may fuss if turned away from the light.
- Stares at faces in close visual range (10–12 inches).
- Signals the need for social stimulation by crying; stops when picked up or put in infant seat close to voices and movement.
- Content to lie on back much of the time.
- Before being picked up, wants to be forewarned by first being touched and talked to.
- Enjoys lots of touching, fondling and holding; but may become fussy with too much stimulation.
- Enjoys "en face" (face to face) position.
- Become less fussy when the television, vacuum or hair dryer are turned on.

DEVELOPMENTAL ALERTS

Check with a health care provider or early childhood specialist if, by one month of age, the infant *does not*:

- Show alarm or "startle" responses to loud noise.
- Suck and swallow with ease.
- Show gains in height, weight and head circumference.
- Grasp with equal strength in both hands.
- Make eye-to-eye contact when awake and being held.
- Quiet soon after being picked up.
- Roll head from side to side when placed on stomach.

ONE TO FOUR MONTHS

It is during these early months that many more of the wonders of infancy begin to unfold. The infant continues to grow at a fast rate. Body systems are fairly well stabilized with body temperature, breathing patterns and heart rate becoming more regular. Longer periods of wakefulness contribute to the infant's personal-social development. Social responsiveness increases as infants begin to practice and to enjoy using their eyes to explore the environment. Infants also begin to find great pleasure in imitating the speech sounds and gestures of others. Increased social awareness allows the infant to begin to establish a sense of trust and emotional attachment to parents and caregivers.

Crying remains the primary way of communicating and of gaining adult attention. However, infants' communication skills soon expand to include body gestures and many non-crying behaviors. Increased strength and voluntary control of muscles contribute to improved motor development. These newly acquired skills are put to constant use throughout the infants' waking hours. During these early months, it must be noted once again, perceptual, cognitive and motor development are closely interrelated and nearly impossible to differentiate. Learning takes place continuously as the infant explores and acquires information about a still new and strange environment.

DEVELOPMENTAL PROFILES AND GROWTH PATTERNS

Growth and Physical Characteristics

- Average length is 20 to 27 inches (50.8–68.6 cm); grows approximately 1 inch (2.54 cm) per month (measured with infant lying on back, from top of the head to bottom of heel, knees straight and foot flexed).
- Weighs an average of 8 to 16 pounds (3.6–7.2 kg); females weighing slightly less than males.
- Gains approximately $1/4$ to $1/2$ lb. per week. (.10–.20 kg)
- Takes approximately 30 to 40 breaths per minute; rate increases significantly during periods of crying or activity.
- Has a normal body temperature ranges from 96.4 to 99.6 F (35.7–37.5 C).
- Head and chest circumference are nearly equal.
- Head circumference increases approximately $3/4$ inch (2 cm) per month until 2 months, then increases $5/8$ inch (1.5 cm) per month until 4 months. Increases are important indications of continued brain growth.
- Has a heart rate (pulse) of approximately 120 to 150 beats per minute at rest.
- Continues to breathe using abdominal (stomach) muscles.
- Posterior fontanel ("soft spot" at the back of the head) closed by the second month.
- Anterior fontanel ("soft spot" on the top of the head) closes to approximately $1/2$ inch (1.3 cm).
- Growth of hair begins to cover scalp.
- Neck is almost non-existent.

- Skin remains sensitive and easily irritated.
- Arms and legs are of equal length, size and shape; easily flexed and extended.
- Legs may appear slightly bowed.
- Feet appear flat with no arch.
- Cries with tears present.

Motor Development

- Reflexive motor behaviors are changing:
    —Tonic neck and stepping reflexes disappear.
    —Rooting and sucking reflexes are well-developed.
    —Swallowing reflex and tongue movements are still immature; continued drooling and inability to move food to the back of the mouth.
    —Landau reflex appears near the middle of this period; when baby is held in a prone (face down) position the head is held upright and legs are fully extended.
- Grasps objects with entire hand; strength insufficient to hold items.
- Holds hands in an open or semi-open position.
- Muscle tone and development equal for boys and girls.
- Muscle strength and control improving; early movements are large and jerky; gradually becoming smoother and purposeful.
- Raises head and upper body on arms when in a prone position.
- Turns head to side when in a supine (face up) position; near the end of this period head is held erect and in line with the body.

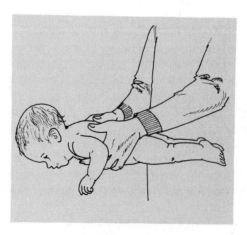

Landau reflex

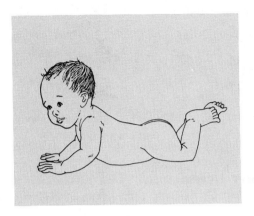

Raises up on arms

- Upper body parts are more active—for example, clasps hands above face, waves arms about, reaches for objects.
- At first, infant rolls from front to back by turning head to one side and allowing trunk to follow; later, infant rolls onto its side. Near the end of this period, infant can roll from front to back to side at will.
- Can be pulled to a sitting position, with considerable head lag and rounded back at the beginning of this period. Later, can be positioned to sit, with minimal head support (hands placed in front for support). Near the end of this period, the infant sits with support, holds head steady and keeps back fairly erect; enjoys sitting in an infant seat or being held on a lap.
- Clasps hands above face; seems fascinated to watch hand (s) approach each other and work together.

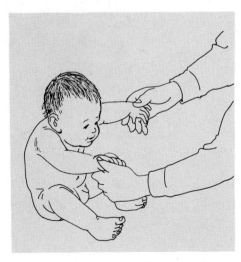

"Held sitting, lumbar curve."

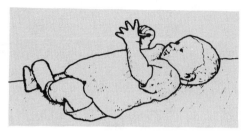

Actively plays with hands

Perceptual-Cognitive Development

- Eyes begin moving together (binocular vision).
- Color vision is present.
- Fixates on a moving object held at 12 inches; smoother visual tracking of objects across 180 degree pathway, vertically and horizontally.
- Continues to gaze in direction of moving objects that disappear.
- Exhibits some sense of size, color, and shape recognition of objects in the immediate environment—for example, recognizes own bottle even when bottle is turned about, thus presenting a different shape.

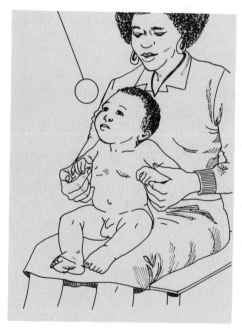

Follows a moving object vertically and horizontally

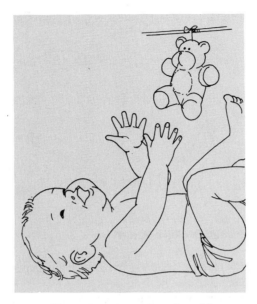

Focuses and reaches for objects

■ Does not search for bottle that falls out of crib or for toy hidden under blanket: "Out of sight, out of mind."
■ Watches hands intently.
■ Moves eyes from one object to another.
■ Focuses eyes on small object and reaches for it; follows hands' movements with eyes.
■ Alternates looking at an object, at one or both hands and then back to the object.
■ Makes same type of gesture as one that was modelled: bye-bye, patting head.
■ Hits at object closest to right or left hand with some degree of accuracy.
■ Correctly localizes the source of a sound.
■ Connects sound and rhythms with movement by moving or jiggling in time to music, singing or chanting.
■ **Discriminates** mother's face from stranger's face when other cues such as voice, touch or smell are also available. (Not clear that this age infant can tell the difference between mother and stranger or even mother and father).
■ Attempts to keep toy in motion by repeating arm or leg movements that started the toy moving in the first place.
■ Begins to mouth objects.

---

discriminates—This is the ability to distinguish or tell the difference between objects or events.

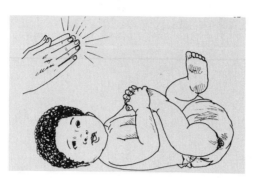

Turns toward sound

Speech and Language Development

- Reacts (stops whimpering, startles, turns head) to sounds such as a voice, rattle of a spoon, ringing of a bell.
- Coordinates looking, vocalizing and body movements when interacting in face-to-face exchanges with parent or caregiver. Can also get an adult to follow infant's lead. In other words, the infant can both follow and lead in keeping a social interaction going.
- Babbles or coos when spoken to or smiled at.
- Produces single vowel sounds (*ah, eh, uh*); also imitates own sounds and vowel sounds produced by others.
- Searches for source of voice (turns head, eyes look for speaker).
- Laughs out loud.

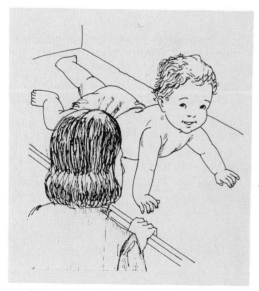

Responds with a social smile

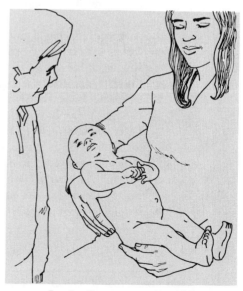

Looks for person speaking

Personal-Social Development

- Uses eyes to imitate, maintain, terminate and avoid interactions—for example, infant turns at will, toward or away from a person or situation.
- Reacts differently to adult voices, may frown or look anxious if voices are loud, angry or unfamiliar.
- Enjoys being held and cuddled at times other than feeding and bedtime.
- Coos, gurgles and squeals when awake.
- Smiles in response to a friendly face or voice.
- Looks for person who is speaking.
- Can entertain self by playing with fingers, hands and toes.
- Enjoys familiar routines, such as being bathed and having diaper changed.
- Delights in play that involves tickling, laughing and gentle poking and jiggling.
- Spends much less time crying.
- Reaches out to familiar persons.
- Recognizes familiar faces and objects, such as father, a bottle; reacts by waving arms and legs and squealing with excitement.
- Stops crying when parent or caregiver comes near.

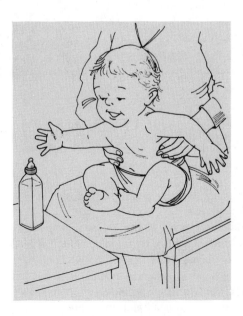

Recognizes and enjoys familiar routines

DAILY ROUTINES—1 TO 4 MONTHS

Eating

- Takes 3 to 5 feedings per day.
- Begins fussing before anticipated feeding times; does not always cry to signal the need to eat.
- Needs only a little assistance in getting nipple to mouth; beginning to help by using own hands to guide nipple.
- Sucks vigorously; may choke on occasion with the vigor and enthusiasm of sucking.
- Becomes impatient if bottle or breast continues to be offered once hunger is satisfied.
- Begins to accept small amounts of solid foods such as mashed banana or cereal when placed well back on tongue. (If food is placed on tip of tongue infant will push it out.)

Bathing, Dressing, Toilet Needs

- Enjoys bath; kicks, laughs and splashes.
- Has one or two bowel movements per day; frequently skips a day.
- Establishing a regular time for bowel movements according to infant's own pattern.

Sleeping

- Often falls asleep for the night soon after the evening feeding.
- Begins to sleep through the night; many babies do not sleep more than 6 hours at a stretch for several more months.
- Averages 14½ to 17 hours of sleep per day; often awake for 2 or 3 periods during the daytime.
- Thumbsucking begins during this period.
- Begins to entertain self before falling asleep—for example, "talks," plays with hands, jiggles crib.

Play and Social Acitivity

- Spends waking periods in physical activity: kicking, turning head from side to side, clasping hands together, grasping objects.
- Becoming "talkative"; vocalizes with delight.
- Likes being talked to and sung to, may cry when the social interaction ends.
- Appears happy when awake and alone (for short periods of time).

DEVELOPMENTAL ALERTS

Check with a health care provider or early childhood specialist if, by four months of age, the infant *does not*:

- Continue to show steady and measurable increases in height, weight and head circumference.
- Smile in response to the smiles of others (the social smile is considered a major and highly significant developmental milestone).
- Follow a moving object with eyes focusing together.
- Bring hands together over mid-chest.
- Turn head to locate sounds.
- Begin to raise head and upper body when placed on stomach.
- Reach for objects or familiar persons.

FOUR TO EIGHT MONTHS

Between four and eight months the infant is developing a wide range of skills and great variability in using his or her body. Infants seem to be busy every waking moment. They manipulate and mouth toys and other objects that come to hand. They "talk" all the time, making vowel and consonent sounds in ever greater variety and complexity. They initiate social interactions and respond to all kinds of cues from others, such as facial expressions, gestures, and the comings and goings of everyone in the infant's world. Infants at this age have been described as both self-contained and sociable. They move easily from spontaneous, self-initiated activity to social activities initiated by others.

DEVELOPMENTAL PROFILES AND GROWTH PATTERNS

Growth and Physical Characteristics

- Gains approximately 1 lb. (.45 kg) per month in weight.
- Doubles original birth weight.
- Gains approximately ½ inch (1.3 cm) in length per month; babies are an average of 27.5 to 29 inches (70–73 cm) long.
- Gains in length and weight are considered normal if they fall between the 30th and 75th percentile on growth charts; below 5 to 10% or over 90 to 95% is cause for concern.
- Head and chest circumferences are nearly equal.
- Head circumference increases approximately ⅜ inch (1 cm) per month until 6 to 7 months, then ³/₁₆ inch (0.5 cm) per month; head circumference should continue to increase steadily, indicating healthy, on-going brain growth.
- Pulse (heart rate) remains approximately 100 to 140 beats per minute; continues to be affected by infant's activity level.
- Breathing continues to be abdominal and ranges from 25 to 50 breaths per minute depending on the amount of stimulation; rate and patterns vary from infant to infant.
- Teeth begin to appear with upper and lower incisors coming in first; gums may be red and swollen. There may also be increased drooling chewing, biting and mouthing of objects.
- Legs may appear bowed; bowing gradually disappears as infant grows older.
- True eye color is established.

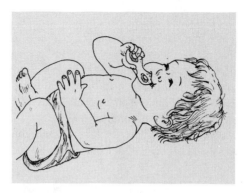

Chews and mouths objects

Motor Development

■ Reflexive behaviors are changing:
—Blinking reflex is well-established
—Sucking reflex becomes voluntary
—Moro reflex disappears
—Parachute reflex appears toward the end of this stage (when held in a prone, horizontal position and lowered suddenly, infant throw out arms as a protective measure).
—Swallowing reflex appears (a more complex form of swallowing that involves tongue movement against the roof of mouth); allows infant to move solid foods from the front of the mouth to the back for swallowing.

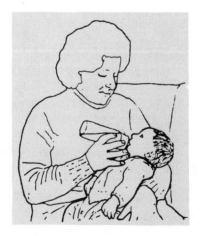

Sucking becomes voluntary

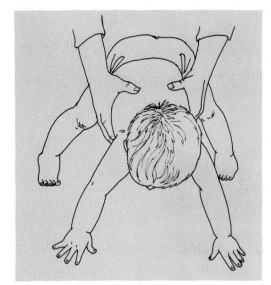

Parachute reflex

- Uses finger and thumb (pincer grasp) to pick up objects.
- Reaches for objects with both arms simultaneously; later reaches with one hand or the other.
- Transfers objects from one hand to the other; grasps object using entire hand (palmar grasp).
- Handles, shakes and pounds objects; puts everything into mouth.
- Holds own bottle.
- Sits alone without support and holds head erect (arms propped forward for support).
- Pulls self into a crawling position by raising up on arms and drawing knees up beneath the body; rocks back and forth, but generally does not move forward.
- Lifts head when placed on back.
- Rolls over from front to back and back to front.
- May accidentally begin scooting backwards when placed on stomach; soon will begin to crawl forward.
- Enjoys being placed in standing position, especially on someone's lap; jumps in place.

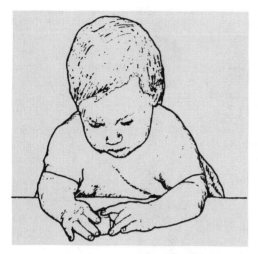

Transfers objects from one hand to the other

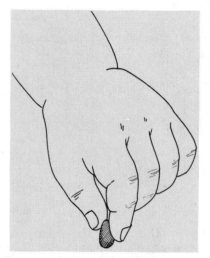

Uses finger and thumb in pincer grasp

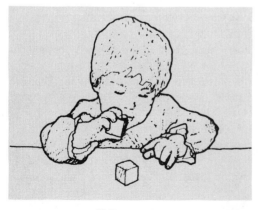

Palmar grasp

Perceptual-Cognitive Development

- Turns toward and locates familiar voices and sounds. (These cues can be used to informally test hearing).
- Focuses eyes on small objects and reaches for them
- Uses hand, mouth and eyes in coordination to explore own body, toys and surroundings.
- Imitates actions such as pat-a-cake, waving bye-bye and playing peek-a-boo.
- Shows fear of falling off high places such as changing table, stairs. Depth perception is clearly evident.
- Looks over side of crib or high chair for objects dropped; delights in repeatedly throwing objects overboard for caregiver to retrieve.
- Searches for toy or food that has been completely hidden under cloth or behind screen; beginning to understand that objects continue to exist even when they cannot be seen. (Piaget refers to this as "object permanence.")
- Handles and explores objects in a variety of ways: visually, turning them around; feeling all surfaces; banging and shaking them.
- Picks up inverted object (in other words, recognizes it's a cup even though it is positioned differently).
- Responds with appropriate actions to specific objects; can slide, crumple, swing, tear, stretch, rub together or place one object inside another according to its characteristics.
- Unable to deal with more than one toy at a time; may either ignore second toy or drop toy already in one hand and focus vision on the new toy.
- Reaches accurately with either hand.
- Plays actively with small toys such as a rattle.
- Bangs objects together playfully; bangs spoon on table.
- Holds small object in one hand while reaching toward another object.
- Continues to take everything to mouth.
- Full attachment to mother or single caregiver. Coincides with growing understanding of "object permanence", the idea that objects exist even when they are no longer visible.

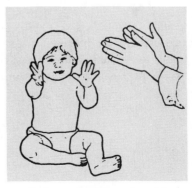

Enjoys playing pat-a-cake

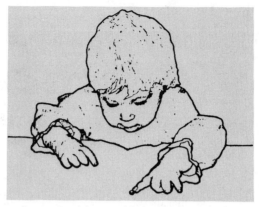

Inspects objects with eyes and hands

Speech and Language Development

- Attends appropriately to familiar words, such as "no-no," "daddy," "go bye-by?"
- Responds to own name.
- Imitates some nonspeech sounds, such as cough, tongue click, lip smacking.
- Produces a full range of vowels and some consonants: *r, s, z, th,* and *w.*
- Responds to variations in the tone of voice of others—anger, playfulness, sadness.
- Expresses emotions such as pleasure, satisfaction and anger by making different sounds.
- "Talks" to toys.
- Babbles by repeating same syllable in a series: *ba, ba, ba.*
- Responds to simple requests: "Wave bye-bye," "Come."
- Makes different responses to vacuum cleaner, phone ringing, dog barking; may cry, whimper, or look toward parent or caregiver for reassurance.

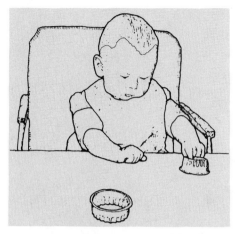

Recognizes inverted object

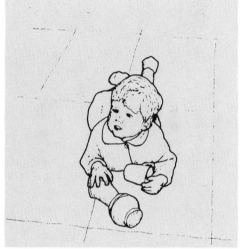

Holds one toy while reaching for another

Personal-Social Development

■ Looks with interest at surroundings; continuously watching people and activities.

■ Developing an awareness of self as a separate individual from others.

■ Becoming more outgoing and social in nature: smiles, coos, reaches out.

■ Can tell the difference between and responds differently to strangers, caretakers, parents, brothers and sisters.

■ Responds differently and appropriately to facial expressions such as frowns, smiles.

■ Imitates facial expressions, actions and sounds made by others.

■ Still friendly toward strangers at the beginning of this stage; later is reluctant to be approached by or left with strangers; exhibits "stranger anxiety."

■ Enjoys being held and cuddled; indicates desire to be picked up by raising arms.

■ Establishes a trust relationship with parents and caregiver if physical and emotional needs are consistently met.

■ Laughs out loud.

■ Becomes upset if toy or other objects are taken away.

■ Seeks attention of parent or caregiver by using body movements, verbalizations, or both.

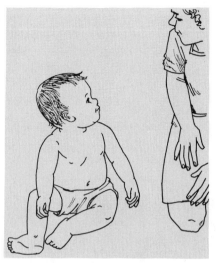

Responds to own name

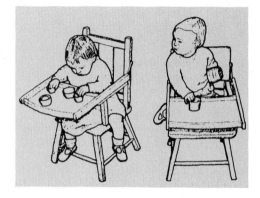

Turns to watch people and activities

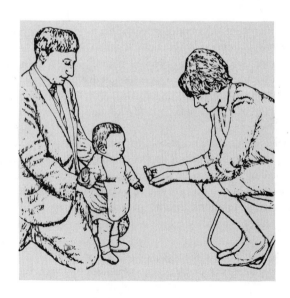

Still friendly with strangers

DAILY ROUTINES—4 TO 8 MONTHS

Eating

- Adjusts feeding times to the family's schedule; usually takes 3 or 4 feedings per day depending upon sleep schedule.
- Shows interest in feeding activities; reaches for cup and spoon while being fed.
- Able to wait half hour or more after awakening for first morning feeding.
- Has less need for sucking; begins to enjoy solid foods if chopped fine.
- Closes mouth firmly or turns head away when hunger is satisfied.

Toileting, Bathing, Dressing

- Enjoys being free of clothes.
- Splashes vigorously with both hands and sometimes feet.
- Hands moving constantly; nothing within reach is safe from being spilled or dashed to floor.
- Pulls off own socks; plays with strings and buttons and velcro closures on clothing.
- Has one bowel movement per day as a general rule.
- Urinates often and in quantity; female infants tend to have longer intervals between wetting.

Sleeping

- Awakens between 6 and 8 a.m.; usually falls asleep soon after evening meal.
- No longer wakens for a late-night feeding.
- Sleeps 11 to 13 hours through the night.
- Takes 2 or 3 naps per day, (great variability among infants).

Play and Social Activity

- Enjoys lying on back; arches back, kicks, stretches legs upwards, grasps feet and brings them to mouth.
- Looks at own hands with interest and delight; may squeal or gaze at them intently.
- Enjoys playing with soft, squeaky toys and rattles; puts them in mouth, bites and chews on them.
- "Talks" happily to self: gurgles, growls, makes high squealing sounds.
- Differentiates between people: lively with those who are familiar, anxious about or ignores others (this is sometimes referred to as a period of "stranger anxiety").
- Likes rhythmic activities: being bounced, jiggled, tossed about gently.

DEVELOPMENTAL ALERTS

Check with a health care provider or early childhood specialist if, by eight months of age, the infant *does not*:

- Show even, steady increase in weight height and head size, (too slow or too rapid growth are both cause for concern).
- Explore own hands and objects placed in hands.
- Hold and shake a rattle.
- Smile, babble and laugh aloud.
- Search for hidden objects.
- Use finger and thumb (pincer grasp) to pick up objects.
- Play games such as "pat-a-cake" and "peek-a-boo".
- Appear interested in new or unusual sounds.
- Reach for and grasp objects.
- Sit alone.
- Begin to eat some solid foods.

EIGHT TO TWELVE MONTHS

Between eight months and one year of age, the infant is gearing up for two major developmental events—walking and talking. These usually begin about the time of the first birthday. The infant is becoming skillful at manipulating small objects and spends a great deal of time practicing by picking up and releasing toys or whatever else is at hand. Infants at this age are also becoming extremely sociable. They find ways to be the center of attention and to get approval and applause from family and friends. When the applause is forthcoming, the infant joins in with unselfconscious delight. The ability to imitate is also developing. It will serve two purposes: to extend social interactions and to help the child learn many new skills and behaviors in the months of rapid development that lie ahead.

DEVELOPMENTAL PROFILES AND GROWTH PATTERNS

Growth and Physical Characteristics

- Gains in height are slower than during the previous months, averaging ½ inch (1.3 cm) per month. Infants reach approximately 1½ times their birth length by their first birthday.
- Weight increases by approximately 1 lb (.45 kg) per month; birth weight is nearly tripled by 1 year of age with infants weighing an average of 21 lbs (9.45 kg).
- Heart rate averages 100 to 140 beats per minute depending on activity.
- Respiration rates vary depending on activity; may range from 20 to 45 breaths per minute.
- Body temperature ranges from 96.4 F. to 99.6 F. (35.7–37.5 C); still affected somewhat by environmental conditions—for example, weather, activity, clothing.
- Head and chest circumference are equal.
- Continues to use abdominal muscles for breathing.
- Anterior fontanel begins to close.
- Approximately 4 upper and 4 lower incisors and 2 lower molars erupt.
- Arm and hands are more developed than feet and legs (cephalo-caudal development); hands appear large in proportion to other body parts.
- Legs may continue to appear bowed.
- Feet appear flat as arch has not yet fully developed.
- Visual acuity is approximately 20/100.

Motor Development

- Reaches with one hand leading in order to grasp an offered object or toy.
- Manipulates objects, transferring them from one hand to the other.
- Explores new objects by poking with one finger.
- Uses deliberate finger and thumb movement (pincer grasp) to pick up small objects, toys and finger foods.
- Stacks objects; also places objects inside one another.
- Releases objects or toys by dropping or throwing; cannot intentionally put an object down.
- Beginning to pull self to a standing position.
- Beginning to stand alone, leaning on furniture for support; moves around objects by side-stepping.
- Sits for indefinite lengths of time; has good balance and can shift positions without losing balance.
- Creeps on hands and knees.
- Crawls up and down stairs.
- Walks with adult support, holding onto adult's hand; may begin to walk alone.
- Grasping objects now under voluntary control.

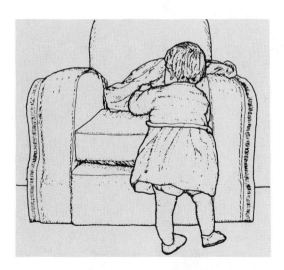

Pulls self to standing

Perceptual-Cognitive Development

- Watches people, objects and activities in the environment.
- Shows awareness of distant objects (15 to 20 feet away) by pointing at them.
- Both eyes working together (referred to as binocular coordination).
- Responds to hearing tests (voice localization); however, loses interest quickly and therefore difficult to test informally.
- Follows simple instructions.
- Reaches for toys out of reach but visible.
- Still takes everything to mouth.
- Continues to drop first item when trying to take three offered items.
- Recognizes the reversal of an object: cup upsidedown is still a cup.
- Plays pat-a-cake.
- Imitates activities such as hitting 2 blocks together.
- Uncovers block hidden by cloth when asked: "Where's the block?"
- Drops toys intentionally and repeatedly; looks in direction of fallen object.
- Shows appropriate use of everyday items: pretends to drink from cup, put on necklace, hug doll, make stuffed animal "walk".
- Shows some sense of spacial relationships: puts block in cup and takes it out when requested to do so.
- Beginning to show an understanding of causality—for example, hands mechanical toy back to adult to have it rewound.
- Shows some awareness of the working relationship of objects: puts spoon in mouth; places cup on saucer; uses brush to smooth hair.
- Searches for partially hidden toy by the end of this period.

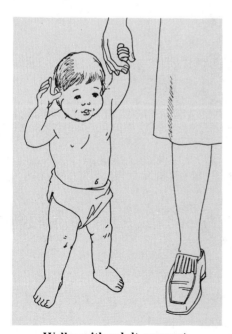

Walks with adult support

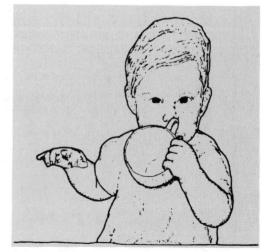

Puts everything in the mouth

Speech and Language Development

- Babbles or jabbers deliberately to get a social interaction started; may shout to attract attention; listens, then shouts again.
- Shakes head for *no* and may nod for *yes*.
- Responds by looking for voice when name is called.
- Babbling in sentence-like sequences that cannot yet be interpreted; followed a bit late by jargon (syllables and sounds with language-like inflection).
- Waves "bye-bye"; pat-a-cakes when asked.
- Says "da-da" and "ma-ma."
- Imitates sounds that are similar to those the baby has already learned to make; will also imitate motor noises, tongue clicks, lip smacking, coughing.
- Enjoys rhymes and simple songs; vocalizes and dances to music.
- Gives a toy or object on request when appropriate gestures accompany the request.

Personal-Social Development

- Exhibits a definite fear or reluctance toward strangers; clings to or hides behind parent or caregiver; resists separating from familiar adult ("stranger anxiety").
- Wants parent or caregiver to be in constant sight.
- Sociable and outgoing; enjoys being near and included in daily activities of family members and caregiver.
- Enjoys novel experiences and opportunities to examine new objects.
- Shows need to be picked up and held by extending arms upward, crying or clinging to adult's legs.
- Begins to be assertive by resisting caregiver's requests; may kick, scream or throw self on the floor.
- Offers toys and objects to others.
- Often becomes attached to a favorite toy or blanket, carrying it about much of the time.
- Upon hearing own name, looks up and smiles at person who is speaking.
- Repeats behaviors that get attention; jabbers continuously.
- Carries out simple directions and requests; understands the meaning of "no."

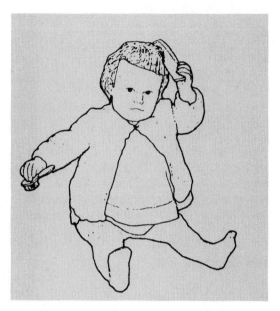

Understands the use of everyday objects

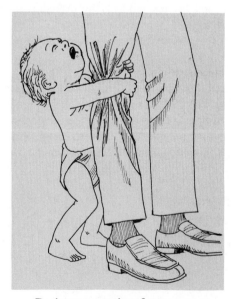

Resists separating from parent

DAILY ROUTINES—8 TO 12 MONTHS

Eating

- Eats three meals a day with midmorning or midafternoon snack of juice or crackers.
- Begins to refuse bottle (if this has not already occurred).
- Has good appetite.
- Enjoys drinking from a cup; holds own cup; will even tilt head backward to get the last bit.
- Begins to eat finger foods; may remove food from mouth, look at it, put it back in.
- Develops certain likes and dislikes for foods.
- Very active; infant's hands may be so busy that a toy is needed for each hand in order to prevent cup or dish from being turned over or food grabbed and tossed about.

Toileting, Bathing, Dressing

- Enjoys bath time; plays with washcloth, soap and water toys.
- Loves to let water drip from sponge or washcloth; sponge-squeezing great sport, too.
- Shows great interest in pulling off hats, taking shoes and socks off.
- Fusses when diaper needs changing; may pull off soiled or wet diaper.
- Cooperates to some degree in being dressed; helps put arm in arm holes, may even extend leg to have pants put on.
- Has one or two bowel movements per day.
- Occasionally dry after a nap.

Sleeping

- Willing to go to bed; may not go to sleep immediately but will play or walk about in crib, then fall asleep on top of covers.
- Sleeps until 6 or 8 o'clock in the morning.
- Plays alone and quietly for 15 to 30 minutes after awakening; then begins to make demanding noises signaling the need to be up and about.
- Plays actively in crib when awake, crib sides must be up and securely fastened.
- Takes one afternoon nap most days.

Play and Social Activities

- Enjoys all gross motor activities: pulling to stand, cruising, standing alone, creeping. Some babies are walking at this point.
- Enjoys putting things on head: basket, bowl, cup, finds this very funny and expects people to notice and laugh.
- Puts objects in and out of each other: pans that nest, pegs in and out of a box.
- Enjoys hiding behind chairs to play "Where's baby?"
- Throws things on floor and expects them to be returned.
- Shows interest in opening and closing doors and cupboards.
- Gives an object to adult on request; expects to have it returned immediately.
- Responds to "no-no" by stopping; on the other hand, the infant may smile, laugh and continue doing what he or she was requested not to do, thus making a game of it.

DEVELOPMENTAL ALERTS

Check with a health care provider or early childhood specialist if, by 12 months of age, the infant *does not*:

- Blink when fast-moving objects approach the eye.
- Begin to cut teeth.
- Imitate simple sounds.
- Follow simple verbal requests: *come, no no, bye bye.*
- Pull to stand.
- Transfer objects from hand to hand.
- Show anxiety toward strangers.
- Interact playfully with parents, caregivers, brothers and sisters.
- Feed self; hold own bottle or cup; pick up and eat finger foods.
- Creep or crawl.

REVIEW QUESTIONS

1. List three characteristics of the newborn infant.
    a.

    b.

    c.

2. List three ways in which it is possible to informally evaluate hearing in an infant who is not yet talking.
    a.

    b.

    c.

3. List three reflexes present in the newborn that should disappear by the time the infant is a year old.
    a.

    b.

    c.

4. List three perceptual-cognitive skills that appear during the first year of life.
    a.

    b.

    c.

TRUE OR FALSE

1. Newborn infants sleep most of the time and are incapable of learning until they can stay awake for one to two hours at a time.

2. The newborn will alert (startle) in response to a loud noise.

3. Crying serves no useful developmental function except to let the infant signal hunger or need to be changed or covered more warmly.

4. An infant's head circumference is measured regularly in order to assess brain growth.

5. Imitation should be discouraged in infants to ensure that they will not grow up to be "copy cats."

6. The healthy infant has nearly tripled its birth weight by one year of age.

7. All normally developing infants crawl on all fours before they walk.

8. The six-month-old who keeps throwing toys out of the crib should be scolded for causing so much work for the parent or caregiver.

9. Developmentally, there is no excuse for nine- or ten-month-old children to be afraid of strangers unless they have previously had a bad experience.

MULTIPLE CHOICE.   Select one item in each of the following groupings that is *not* seen in the majority of infants in the age category listed.

1. Birth to 28 days
    a. cries without tears.
    b. synchronizes body movements to speech patterns of parent or caregiver.
    c. shows need to be picked up by extending arms.

2. One to four months
    a. waves bye-bye, plays pat-a-cake upon request.
    b. babbles or coos when spoken to or smiled at.
    c. TNR (tonic neck reflex) and stepping reflex disappear.

3. Four to eight months
    a. shows full attachment to mother or major caregiver.
    b. expresses emotions such as pleasure, anger and distress by making different kinds of sounds.
    c. sees outlines and shapes of nearby objects but cannot focus on distant objects.

4. Eight months to one year
    a. usually sleeps through the night.
    b. cuts several teeth.
    c. a vocabulary of at least 50 words.

Chapter 4

The Toddler

TWELVE TO EIGHTEEN MONTHS

The toddler is a dynamo, full of unlimited energy and enthusiasm. Only moderate changes occur in growth during this stage. There are, however, significant changes in other developmental areas. The toddler period begins with the limited abilities of an infant and ends with the relatively sophisticated skills of a young child.

Improvements in motor skills continue. This allows toddlers to move about on their own, and to explore and test their surroundings. Rapid speech and language development contributes to the toddler's thinking and learning abilities. **Defiance** and negative responses become commomplace near the end of this stage. The toddler begins to assert independence as a way of gaining autonomy (a sense of self as separate and self-managed) and some degree of control over parents and caregivers.

---

defiance—*Refusal to do what has been requested is defiance.*

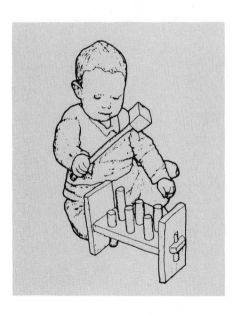

The toddler is full of unlimited energy.

DEVELOPMENTAL PROFILES AND GROWTH PATTERNS

Growth and Physical Characteristics

- Rate of growth is considerably slower during this period.
- Height increases approximately 2.5 to 3 inches (6.4–7.6 cm) per year to an average of 26 to 28 inches (66–71 cm); height is approximately 1½ times the original length at birth.
- Weighs approximately 21 to 27 pounds (9.5–12.2 kg) gains ¼ to ½ pounds (0.1–0.2 kg) per month; is approximately three times heavier than original birth weight.
- Respiration rate is approximately 24 to 30 and stable; varies with emotional state and activity.
- Heart beats approximately 80 to 120 times per minute.
- Blood pressure is approximately 96/64.
- Head size increases slowly; grows approximately ½ inch (1.3 cm) every six months.
- Chest circumference is larger than head circumference.
- Rapid eruption of teeth; approximately 6 to 10 new teeth appear.
- Requires approximately 1300 calories daily.
- Anterior fontanel is almost completely closed.
- Bones of skull begin to thicken.
- Legs may appear bowed.
- Body shape changes; takes on more adult-like appearance; still top heavy, abdomen protruding.
- Visual acuity is approximately 20/60.

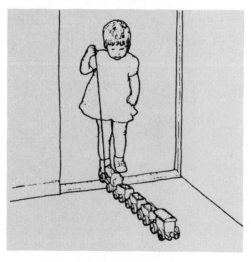

Enjoys pushing or pulling toys

Motor Development

- Crawls skillfully and quickly.
- Stands alone with feet spread apart and arms extended for support.
- Gets to feet by self.
- Begins to walk unassisted near the end of this period; falls often; not always able to maneuver around obstacles such as furniture or toys.
- Uses furniture to lower self to floor; collapses backwards into a sitting position or falls forward on hands and then sits.
- Voluntarily releases an object.
- Enjoys pushing or pulling toys while walking.
- Repeatedly picks up objects and throws them.
- Opens and looks inside a box.
- Attempts to run or "toddle"; has difficulty stopping and usually drops to the floor.
- Crawls backwards down stairs.
- Carries toys from place to place.
- Enjoys using crayons or markers to scribble.
- Helps feed self; enjoys holding spoon and drinking from a glass or cup; not always accurate at getting utensils into mouth; frequent spills.
- Helps to turn pages of a book.
- Stacks 2 to 4 objects on top of one another.

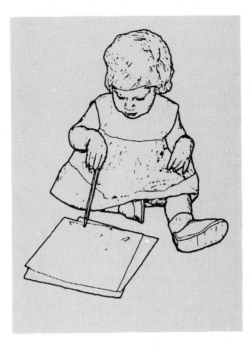

Enjoys scribbling

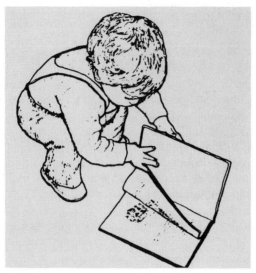

Turns pages of books

Perceptual-Cognitive Development

■ Enjoys object-hiding activities:
—Early in this period the child always searches in the same location for a hidden object (if child has watched the hiding of the object).
—Later in this period, the child will search in several locations; (again, only if child has watched the hiding of the object).

■ Passes toy to hand on other side of midline (center of the body) when offered a second object or toy.

■ Manages 3 to 4 objects by setting an object aside (on lap or floor) when presented with a new toy.

■ Seldom puts toys in mouth.

■ Enjoys looking at pictures in books.

■ Demonstrates understanding of functional relationships (objects that belong together):
—Puts spoon in bowl and then uses spoon as in eating.
—Places cup on saucer and sips from cup.
—Tries to make doll stand up.

■ Shows or offers toy for another person to look at.

■ Names everyday objects.

■ Places nine small blocks in a container.

■ Puts all pegs in a six-peg board (large pegs).

■ Puts small item (raisin, Cheerio) in and dumps it out of a bottle.

■ Places 3 geometric shapes in large form board.

■ Makes balanced tower of 3 small blocks

■ Attempts to activate mechanical objects if child has seen someone else make them work.

■ Responds with some facial movement but cannot truly imitate facial expressions.

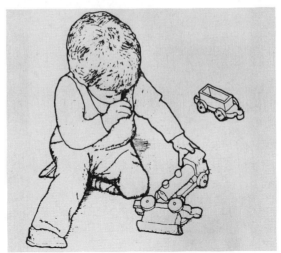

Links toys in functional relationships

Speech and Language Development

- Produces considerable "jargon": words and sounds put together into speech-like (inflected) patterns.
- "Holophrastic" speech: one word conveys an entire thought; meanings depend upon the inflection.
- Follows simple directions: "Give daddy the cup."
- When asked, will point to familiar persons, animals, and toys.
- Identifies three body parts if someone names them: "Show me your nose." " . . . your toe." " . . . your ear."
- Produces some two word phrases: "More cookie," "Daddy bye-bye."
- Indicates a few desired objects and activities by name: "Bye-bye," "cookie"; verbal request is often accompanied by an insistent gesture.
- Responds to simple questions with "yes" or "no" and appropriate head movements.
- Speech is 25% **intelligible**.
- Locates familiar objects on request (if objects are in locations the child knows about).
- Uses 5 to 50 words; typically these are words that refer to animals, food and toys.
- Hands mechanical toy to adult as a "request" to have it wound.
- Hands objects to others as a way of initiating social interaction.
- Uses gestures such as pointing or pulling to direct adult attention.
- Enjoys rhymes and tries to join in.
- Seems aware of the reciprocal (back and forth) aspects of conversational exchanges; some turn-taking in other kinds of vocal exchanges such as making and imitating sounds.

---

intelligible—When language is intelligible, it is capable of being understood by others.

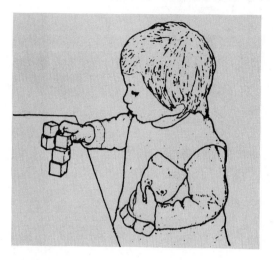

Makes balanced tower of two to three blocks

Personal-Social Development

- Usually friendly toward others; less wary of strangers.
- Enjoys singing songs along with an adult.
- Helps pick up and put away toys.
- Engages in solitary play (plays alone) for short lengths of time.
- Enjoys being held and read to.
- Often imitates adult's actions in play.
- Enjoys adult attention; still likes to know that an adult is near.
- Recognizes self in mirror.
- Enjoys the companionship of other children but does not play cooperatively.
- Beginning to assert independence; often refuses to cooperate with daily routines that once were enjoyable; resists getting dressed, putting on shoes, eating, taking a bath.
- May have a tantrum when things go wrong or if overly frustrated.
- Exceedingly curious about people and surroundings; needs to be watched carefully to prevent getting into dangerous situations.

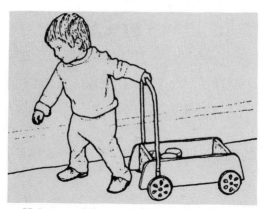

Helps to pick up and put away toys

DEVELOPMENTAL ALERTS

Check with a health care provider or early childhood specialist if, by 18 months of age, the child *does not*:

- Attempt to talk or repeat words.
- Understand some new words.
- Respond to simple questions with "yes," "no."
- Walk alone (or with very little help).
- Exhibit a variety of emotions: anger, delight, fear.
- Show interest in pictures.
- Recognize self in mirror.
- Attempt self-feeding: hold own cup to mouth and drink.

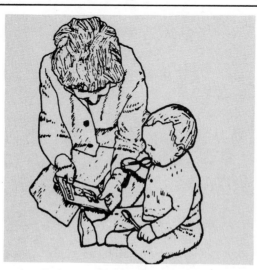

Enjoys having adult near

ONE AND ONE-HALF – TWO YEARS

DEVELOPMENTAL PROFILES AND GROWTH PATTERNS

Growth and Physical Development

- Weight is now approximately four times the original weight at birth; toddler weighs nearly 26 to 32 pounds (11.8–14.5 kg); gains ¼ to ½ pound (0.1–0.2 kg) per month.
- Height is nearly one-half of approximate adult height; grows approximately 2.5 inches (6.4 cm) during the next six months. Average height is 32 to 33 inches (81–84 cm).
- Eruption of teeth is nearly complete; second molars appear for a total of 20 teeth.
- Head circumference increases slowly by 1/2 inch (1.3 cm) over the next six months.
- Heart rate (pulse) is 80 to 110.
- Respirations are approximately 20 to 35 breaths per minute.

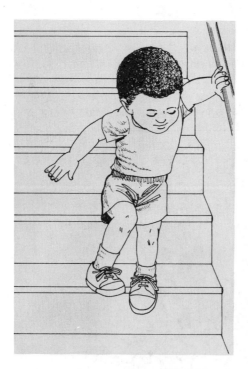

Walks down stairs holding onto railing or adult's hand

Motor Development

- Walks unassisted; maneuvers around objects on floor.
- Runs with confidence; seldom falls; moves quickly from one place to another.
- Walks backwards.
- Walks up or down stairs by holding onto a railing or adult's hand; climbs with both feet on the same step at a time.
- Carries large objects while walking.
- Bends down to pick up toys without falling over.
- Jumps up and down but often falls.
- Climbs on chair, turns around and sits down.
- Sits by self in child-size chair.
- Feeds self; carefully places spoon in mouth.
- Enjoys pouring and filling activities: sand, water
- Stacks 4 to 6 objects one on top of another.
- Scribbles vigorously with crayons or markers; scribbling is more controlled.
- Opens doors using doorknob.
- Uses feet (on pavement) to move small, wheeled riding toys forward.
- Bowel training often achieved.
- Eyes turn inward, equally, (convergence) as an object is brought close to the face. (Can be used to informally test muscle development of the eyes.)

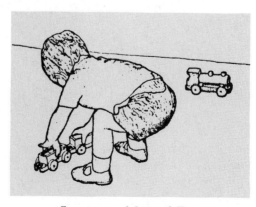

Squats to pick up fallen toy

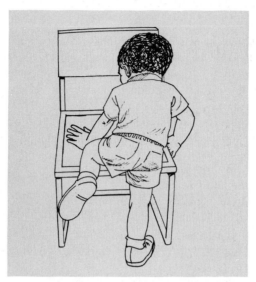

Climbs up into adult chair

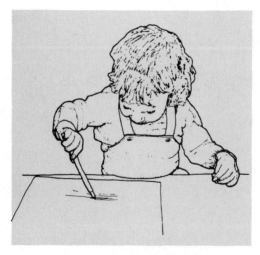

Scribbling is more deliberate

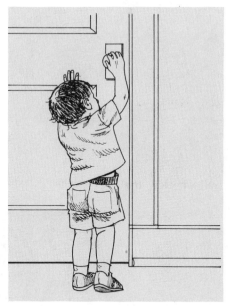

Opens doors using doorknob

Perceptual-Cognitive Development

- Finds an object after it is hidden in one place and then another; looks in last hiding place first and retraces course of earlier moves.
- Watches the course of a small ball, such as a tennis ball; will go and get it.
- Shows understanding of a potential problem; righting a carton of milk before it falls over, for example.
- No longer takes toys to mouth.
- When presented with a variety of objects will look for and put in place those that go together; will use objects in appropriate sequences.
    —Puts cup on saucer, looks for spoon, finds it, pretends to stir; then sips.
    —Puts doll in cradle, finds blanket, covers doll, rocks doll.
- Places 10 small blocks in a container.
- Places 6 square pegs in peg board.
- Builds tower of 4 to 6 small blocks.
- Knows where familiar persons should be; notes their absence.
- Tries to make mechanical toys work without a demonstration.
- Echoes significant, or the last words, that were spoken by someone else.

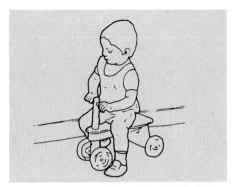

Uses feet to propel small wheeled toys

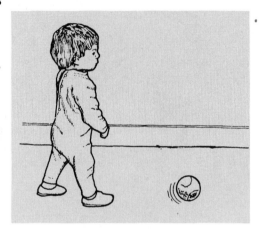

Watches and retrieves rolling ball

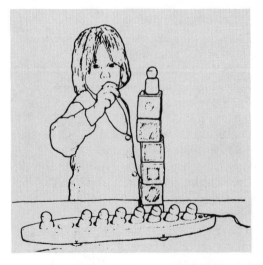

Builds tower of four to six blocks

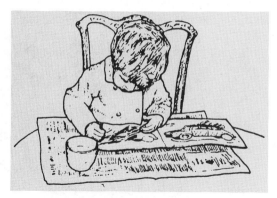

Names familiar objects in books

Speech and Language Development

- Speaks 50 to 300 different words; names almost everything in familiar surroundings.
- Follows directions about placing one item in or on another: "Put the sweater on the bed!" " . . . in the drawer."
- Refers to own self as "me" or sometimes "I" rather than by name: "Me go bye-bye", not "Baby go bye-bye."
- Uses some plurals.
- Asks "What's that?" and "Why?" repeatedly.
- Enjoys stories about self and family.
- Names familiar objects while leafing through a book.
- Speech as much as 65% intelligible.
- Understands most simple directions and questions, especially when accompanied by gestures.
- Uses the words "please" and "thank you" if this is a part of family practice.
- Sings along with familiar tunes.

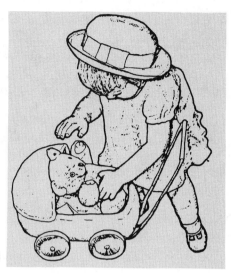

Enjoys make-believe

Personal-Social Development

- Affectionate; offers hugs and kisses.
- Often defiant; says "No" in response to many requests.
- Shows tremendous curiosity; gets into everything, requires constant supervision.
- Watches and imitates the play of other children; seldom joins in.
- Shows increased independence; insists on trying to do many things without help: put on socks, hold own glass.
- Alternates between clinging to parents and caregivers or resisting them.
- Plays well alone; initiates own activities much of the time.
- Eager for adult attention, especially if nearby children are getting the adult's attention.
- Enjoys simple make-believe and role-play activities; dressing up, pretending to pour tea.
- May offer toys to other children, but is usually possessive of playthings; hoards toys.

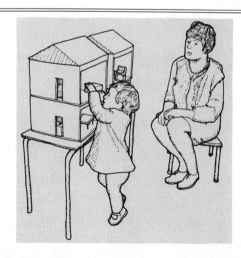

Protective of possessions

DAILY ROUTINES — THE TODDLER (ONE – TWO YEARS)

Eating

- Has a decreased appetite; lunch is often the preferred meal of the day.
- Sometimes described as a finicky or fussy eater; may go on food jags; neither requires, nor wants, a large amount of food.
- Occasionally holds food in mouth without swallowing it; usually indicates child does not need or want any more to eat.
- Uses spoon with some degree of skill (if hungry and interested in eating).
- Has good control of cup: lifts it up, drinks from it, sets it down, holds with one hand.
- Helps feed self; some two-year-olds can feed self independently; others need help.

Bathing, Dressing, Toilet Needs

- Tries to wash self; plays with washcloth and soap.
- Takes off own shoes, stockings, some pants; attempts to dress self, often with little success: tries to put both feet into one pant leg, puts shirt on backwards or upside down.
- Helps when being dressed; puts arm in armhole, lifts feet to have socks put on.
- Lets parent or caregiver know when diaper or pants are soiled or wet.
- Begins to gain some control of bowels and bladder; complete control often not achieved until around age three. Bowel training can begin around twelve months; control is often achieved by eighteen months. Begins some bladder control after eighteen months.

Sleeping

- Falls asleep around 8 or 9 p.m.; however, will often fall asleep at dinner if nap has been missed.
- Makes many requests at bedtime for stuffed toys, a book or two, a special blanket.
- Has some problems going to sleep; overflow of energy shows itself in bouncing and jumping, calling for mother, demanding a drink, insisting on being taken to the bathroom, singing, making and remaking bed, all of which seem to be ways of "winding down."

Play and Social Activity

- Developing a strong sense of property rights; "mine" is heard frequently. Sharing is difficult, hoards toys and other items.
- Enjoys helping, but gets into "trouble" when left alone: smears toothpaste, tries on lipstick, empties dresser drawers.
- Enjoys talking about pictures; likes repetition, as in *Drummer Hoff, Mr. Bear, Dr. Seuss*.
- Enjoys walks; stops frequently to look at things (rocks, gum wrappers, insects); squats to examine them; much dawdling with no real interest in getting any place in particular.
- Still plays alone (solitary play) most of the time, though showing interest in other children, lots of watching; parallel play once in awhile but no cooperative play as yet (exception may be children who have spent considerable time in group care).
- At bedtime needs door left slightly ajar with light on in another room; seems to feel more secure, better able to settle down.
- Continues naps; naps too long or too late will interfere with bedtime.
- Wakes up slowly from nap; cannot be hurried or rushed into any activity at this time.

DEVELOPMENTAL ALERTS

Check with a health care provider or early childhood specialist if, by 30 months, the child does not:

- Verbalize needs and desires.
- Speak in 2 to 3 word phrases.
- Follow a series of two simple commands.
- Enjoy being read to.
- Avoid bumping into objects.
- Climb up and down stairs holding caregiver's hand.
- Throw a ball.
- Chew food; feed self small bites of fruits, meat.
- Help take off own clothes, shoes and socks.

REVIEW QUESTIONS

1. List three motor skills or physical characteristics of the toddler.
    a.

    b.

    c.

2. List three ways in which the toddler may begin to assert independence.
    a.

    b.

    c.

3. List three perceptual-cognitive skills displayed by most toddlers.
    a.

    b.

    c.

TRUE OR FALSE

1. Chest circumference is greater than head circumference.

2. Follows three-step directions by the eighteenth month.

3. Some toddlers are trained to use the toilet for bowel movements by 24 months.

4. Toddlers should be punished for constantly getting into things.

5. Toddlers need constant adult supervision.

6. Toddlers sometimes go on "food jags."

7. Toddlers' appetite increases significantly as compared to infants.

8. Toddlers should be expected to share toys, food, books.

MULTIPLE CHOICE   Select one or more correct answers from the lists below.

1.   Between 12 and 18 months most toddlers
     a.   will get 6 to 10 new teeth.
     b.   are crawling skillfully and many are walking.
     c.   have no way of getting down stairs by themselves.

2.   Which of the following are *not* characteristic of most toddlers' communication skills?
     a.   talking jargon
     b.   using holophrastic speech
     c.   talking in complete sentences

3.   Most toddlers
     a.   are less hesitant to go to strangers than they were in later infancy.
     b.   always play cooperatively, never alone.
     c.   should be taught to use blunt scissors.

4.   It is reasonable to expect most toddlers to
     a.   use a spoon with full control.
     b.   take off own shoes and stockings.
     c.   catch a small ball.

5.   Which of the following best describe the toddler period?
     a.   full of energy and enthusiasm
     b.   frequent negative responses related to independence
     c.   eager to explore and test their surroundings

Chapter 5

The Preschooler

Constant motion, eagerness, curiosity and joy of life characterize the healthy preschool-age child. During these years, abilities in all developmental areas undergo rapid change and expansion. Motor skills are being perfected. Creativity and imagination come into everything from dramatic play to art work to story-telling. Vocabulary and intellectual skills expand rapidly, allowing the child to express ideas, solve problems and plan ahead. Preschool children strongly believe in their own opinions. At the same time, they are developing some sense of the needs of others and some degree of control over their own behavior. Throughout the preschool years they strive for independence, yet they need continual reassurance that an adult is available to give assistance, to comfort or to rescue them if need be.

THE THREE-YEAR-OLD

DEVELOPMENTAL PROFILES AND GROWTH PATTERNS

Earlier conflicts, centered around struggles for independence, become fewer as children enter their third year of life. They are interested in cooperating and in accepting adult's directions. There is also an effort to delay gratification; in other words, they have less need to have what they want "right now." Furthermore, three-year-olds appear to love life. They have an irrepressible urge to find out about everything in their immediate world.

Growth and Physical Development

- Growth is slow and even.
- Height increases 2 to 3 inches (5–7.6 cm) per year; average height is 38 to 40 inches (96.5–101.6 cm) or nearly double the child's original birth length.
- Adult height can be predicted from measurements of height at 3 years of age; males are 53% of their adult height, females 57%.
- Gains 3 to 5 pounds (1.4–2.3 kg) per year; weighs an average of 30 to 38 pounds (13.6–17.3 kg).
- Heart rate (pulse) averages 90–110 beats per minute.
- Respiratory rate is 20–30 depending on activity level; child continues to breath abdominally.
- Blood pressure reading is 84–90/60.

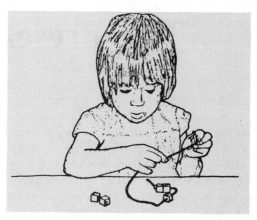

Appearance becoming more adult-like

- Temperature reading averages 96 to 99.4 F. (35.5–37.4 C); is affected by activity, environmental conditions and illness.
- Growth of legs is more rapid than arms giving the three-year-old a taller, thinner, adult-like appearance.
- Circumference of head and chest are equal; head-size is in better proportion to the rest of the body.
- Neck lengthens as "baby fat" disappears.
- Posture is more erect; abdomen no longer protrudes and is smaller.
- Still appears slightly knock-kneed.
- Has a full set of "baby" teeth.
- Needs to consume approximately 1300 calories daily.
- Visual acuity is approximately 20/40 using the Snellen E chart.

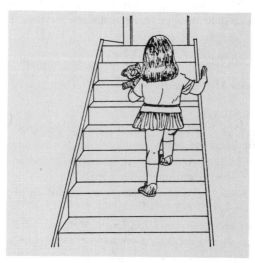

Walks up and down stairs using alternating feet.

Motor Development

- Walks up and down stairs independently, using alternating feet; may jump from bottom step, landing on both feet.
- Can balance momentarily on one foot.
- Hops on one foot.
- Kicks a large ball.
- Feeds self without assistance.
- Jumps in place.
- Pedals a small tricycle or wheeled toy.
- Throws a ball overhand.
- Catches a bounced ball with both arms extended.
- Enjoys swinging on a swing.
- Shows improved control of crayons or markers when drawing; uses vertical, horizontal and circular motions.
- Holds crayon or marker between first two fingers and thumb (tripod grasp), not in a fist as earlier.
- Turns pages of a book one at a time.
- Enjoys building structures with wooden blocks.
- Builds a tower of seven or more blocks.
- Enjoys playing with clay; pounds, rolls and squeezes it.

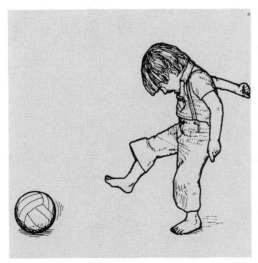

Kicks a large ball.

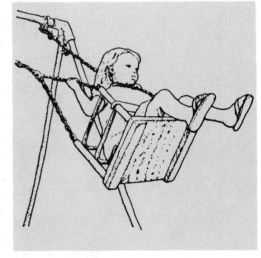

Enjoys swinging on a swing

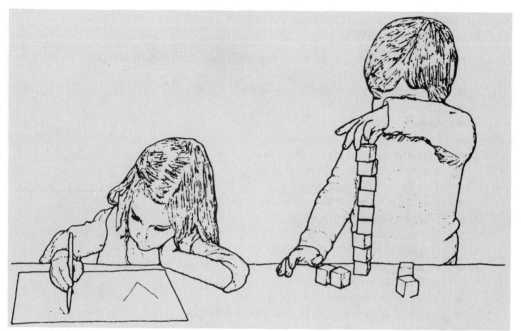

Holds marker in tripod grasp   **Builds tower of seven or more blocks**

- Carries a container of liquid, such as a cup of milk or bowl of water without much spilling; pours liquid from a pitcher into another container.
- Manipulates large buttons and zippers on clothing.
- Washes and dries hands; brushes own teeth.
- Achieves complete bladder control during this time.

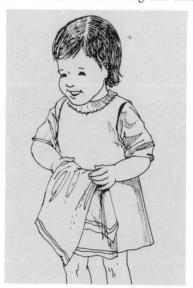

Washes and dries hands.

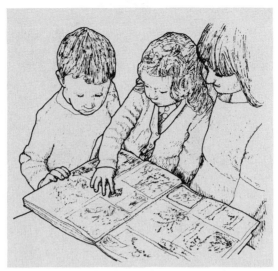

May "read" to others or explain pictures.

Perceptual and Cognitive Development

■ Listens attentively to age-appropriate stories.

■ Makes relevant comments during stories, especially to stories that relate to home and family events.

■ Likes to look at books and may "read" to others or explain pictures.

■ Enjoys stories with riddles, guessing and "suspense" (*The Noisy Book*).

■ Points with 70% accuracy to correct pictures when given sound-alike words: *keys-cheese; fish-dish; mouse-mouth.*

■ Enjoys story books that give real information; already boys are showing preference for stories about machinery.

■ Plays realistically:
　　—Feeds doll, puts it down for nap, covers it up.
　　—Hooks truck and trailer together, loads truck, drives away making motor noises.

■ Places 8 to 10 round pegs in peg board, or 6 round and 6 square blocks in form board.

■ Draws circle, square and some letters.

■ Understands triangle, circle, square; can point to requested shape.

■ Sorts objects logically on the basis of design, shape or color; however, chooses color or size predominantly as basis for classification.

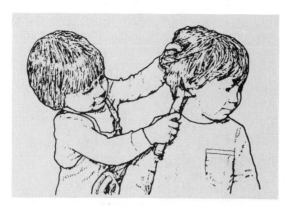

Plays realistically. Pretending to examine playmate's ear.

- Shows understanding of basic size-shape comparisons 80% of the time; for example, will indicate which is bigger when shown tennis and golf balls; also understands smaller of the two.
- Names and matches primary colors: red, yellow, blue
- Makes horizontal train of cubes in imitation of another's model
- Places blocks to make a bridge
- Estimates "how many" in sets of 1 to 4 and sometimes 1 to 5.
- Counts objects out loud
- Chooses picture that has "more": cars, planes or kittens
- Shows some understanding of duration of time by using phrases such as "all the time," "all day," "for two days"; continues to show some confusion: "I didn't take a nap tomorrow."

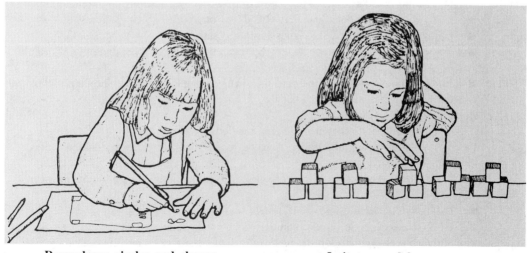

Reproduces circles and shapes   **Imitates models**

Speech and Language

- Talks about known objects, events and people not present: "Jerry has a pool in his yard."
- Talks about the actions of others: "Daddy is mowing the grass."
- Adds information to what has just been said in a conversation: "Yeah, and then he grabbed it back."
- Answers simple questions appropriately.
- Asks increasing numbers of questions, particularly about location and identity of objects and people.
- Uses an increasing number of speech forms that keep conversation going: "What did he do next?"
- Calls attention to self, objects, or events in the environment: "Watch my helicopter fly."
- Promotes the behavior of others: "Let's jump in the water; You go first."
- Asks for desired objects or assistance.
- Joins in social interaction rituals: "Hi," "Bye," "Please."
- Comments about objects and ongoing events: "There's a house," "The tractor's pushing a boat."
- Vocabulary has grown to 300 to 1000 words.
- Recites nursery rhymes, sings songs.
- Speech is 80% intelligible.
- Produces expanded noun phrases: ". . . big, brown dog";
- Produces verbs with "ing" endings; uses "-s" to indicate more than one.
- Uses the preposition "in."
- Indicates negatives by inserting "no" or "not" before a simple noun or verb phrase, "Not baby."
- Answers "What are you doing?" "What is this?" and "Where?" questions dealing with familiar objects and events.

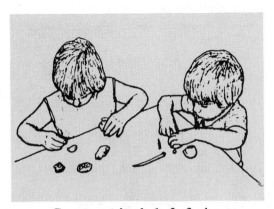

Counts out loud: 1, 2, 3, 4 . . .

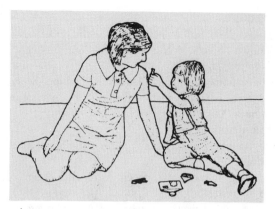

Answers questions about familiar objects and events

Personal-Social Development

- Seems to understand taking turns, but not always willing to do so.
- Friendly; laughs frequently; is eager to please.
- Occasional nightmares and fears of the dark, monsters or fire.
- Joins in simple games and group activities, sometimes hesitantly.
- Often talks to self.
- Uses objects symbolically in play; block of wood may be pushed as a truck, aimed as a gun, used as a ramp.
- Observes other children playing; may join in for a short time; often plays parallel to other children.
- Defends toys and other possessions; may become physically aggressive at times by grabbing a toy away, hitting another child, hiding toys.
- Engages in make-believe play alone and with other children.
- Shows affection toward children who are younger or children who get hurt.
- Sits and listens to stories up to ten minutes at a time; does not bother other children listening to story and resents being bothered.
- May continue to have a special security blanket, stuffed animal or toy for comfort.

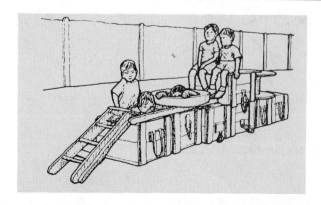

Engages in make-believe

DAILY ROUTINES—THREE-YEAR-OLDS

Eating

■ Appetite fairly good; prefers small servings. Likes only a few cooked vegetables; eats almost everything else.
■ Feeds self independently if hungry. Uses spoon in semi-adult fashion; may even spear with fork.
■ Dawdles over food when not hungry.
■ Can pour milk and juice and serve individual portions from a serving dish with some prompts ("Fill it up to the line"; "Take only two spoonsful.")
■ Begins to drink a great deal of milk. (Must be sure child does not fill up on milk to the exclusion of other needed foods.)

Bathing, Dressing, Toileting

■ Does a fair job of washing self in bath tub; still resists getting out of tub.
■ Takes care of own toilet needs during the daytime (boys, especially, may continue to have pants-wetting accidents).
■ Sleeps through the night without wetting the bed; some children are in transition—some days or even weeks they are dry, then may again experience night-wetting for a period.
■ Child still more skilled at undressing than dressing self, though capable of putting on some articles of clothing.
■ Becomes more skilled at manipulating buttons, large snaps, and zippers.

Sleeping

■ Usually sleeps 10 to 12 hours at night, waking up about 7 or 8 a.m.; some children are awake much earlier.
■ May no longer take an afternoon nap; continues to benefit from a quiet time on bed.
■ Can get self ready for bed. Has given up many earlier bedtime rituals; still need a bedtime story or song and tucking-in.
■ May begin to have dreams that cause the child to awaken.
■ Night wanderings may occur; quiet firmness is needed in returning child to his or her own bed, not parents' bed.

Play and Social Activity

■ The "me too" age; wants to be included in everyting.
■ Spontaneous group play for short periods of time; very social; beginning to play cooperatively.
■ May engage in arguments with other children; adults should allow children to settle their own disagreements unless physical harm is threatened.
■ Loves dress-up, dramatic play that involves every day work activities. Strong sex-role stereotypes: "Boys can't be nurses."
■ Responds well to options rather than commands. "Do you want to put your nightgown on before or after the story?"
■ Sharing still difficult, but seems to understand the concept.

DEVELOPMENTAL ALERTS

Check with a health care provider or early childhood specialist if, by three years of age, the child *does not*:

- Have intelligible speech most of the time.
- Understand and follow simple commands and directions.
- Give own name.
- Enjoy playing near other children.
- Use 3 to 4 word sentences.
- Ask questions.
- Stay with an activity for 5 to 10 minutes.
- Jump in place without falling.
- Balance on one foot.
- Help with dressing self.

THE FOUR-YEAR-OLD

Four-year-olds are bundles of energy. They seem to be engaged in non-stop activity during every waking moment. Bouts of stubbornness and arguments may be frequent between child and parent or caregiver. It is a time of constantly testing limits in order to practice self-confidence and firm up a growing need for independence. At four, many children are loud, boisterous, even belligerent. They try adults' patience with their silly talk and silly jokes, their constant chatter and endless questions. At the same time, four-year-olds have many lovable qualities. They are enthusiastic, try hard to be helpful, have lively imaginations, and can plan ahead to some extent: "When we get home, I'll make you some toast."

DEVELOPMENTAL PROFILES AND GROWTH PATTERNS

Growth and Physical Characteristics

- Gains an average of 4 to 5 pounds (1.8–2.3 kg) per year; weighs an average of 32 to 40 pounds (14.5–18.2 kg).
- Grows 2 to 2.5 inches (5.0–6.4 cm) in height per year; is approximately 40 to 45 inches (101.6–114 cm) tall.
- Heart rate (pulse) averages 90–110 beats per minute.
- Respiratory rate ranges from 20–30 varying with activity and emotional level.
- Body temperature ranges from 98 to 99.4 F (36.6–37.4 C).
- Blood pressure remains at 84/60.
- Head circumference is usually not measured after age three.
- Requires approximately 1700 calories daily.
- Hearing acuity can be assessed by child's correct usage of sounds and language.
- Visual acuity is 20/30 as measured on the Snellen E chart.

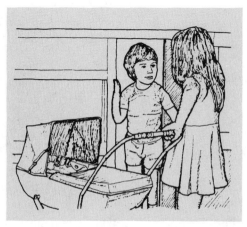

Affectionate toward younger children

Motor Development

- Walks on a straight line.
- Hops on one foot.
- Pedals and steers a tricycle or wheeled toy with confidence and skill; turns corners, avoids obstacles.
- Climbs ladders, steps, trees, play ground equipment.
- Jumps over objects five or six inches high or from a step; lands with both feet together.
- Runs, starts, stops and moves around obstacles with ease.
- Throws a ball overhand.
- Builds a tower with ten or more blocks using the dominant hand.
- Forms shapes and objects out of clay: cookies, snakes, animals.
- Reproduces shapes and letters O, H, T, and V.
- Holds a crayon or marker using a tripod grasp.
- Paints and draws with deliberateness.
- Crosses legs when sitting on the floor.
- Becomes more accurate at hitting nails and pegs with hammer.
- Threads small beads on a string.

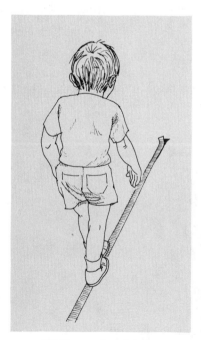

Walks a straight line

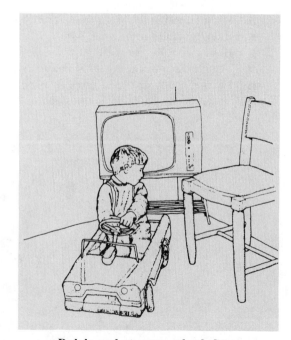

Pedals and steers a wheeled toy

Perceptual and Cognitive Development

- Stacks 5 graduated cubes from largest to smallest.
- Builds a pyramid of 6 blocks.
- Can tell if paired words are the same or different in sound: *sheet/feet, ball/wall*.
- Places lower and upper case letters in form board.
- Near the end of this period, child may name about 75% of capital letters; can also write a few capital letters; may print own name.
- Recognizes several printed words.
- Some children are beginning to read very simple books with only a few words per page and many pictures.
- Interested in alphabet books.
- Likes stories about how things grow and how things operate.
- Delights in words, plays on words, creates silly language.
- Understands the concepts of "tallest," "biggest," "same," and "more"; selects the picture that has the "most houses" in it or the "biggest dogs."
- Identifies the number of pennies or chips from one to four by looking at the groups.
- Rote counts to 20.
- Counts out a requested set of objects (1 to 7) when given a larger group of objects.
- Matches a set of 3 objects by pointing to the correct numeral.
- Has a clear understanding of the sequence of daily events: "When we get up in the morning, we get dressed, have breakfast, brush our teeth and go to school."

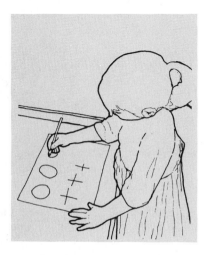

Reproduces shapes and letters

Speech, and Language

- Uses the prepositions "on," "in," and "under."
- Uses possessives consistently: "hers," "theirs," "baby's."
- Uses "can't" and "don't" as well as "cannot" and "do not" to mark negatives.
- Answers "Whose?" "Who?" "Why?" and "How many?"
- Produces elaborate sentence structures: "The cat ran under the house before I could see what color it was."
- Speech is 95% intelligible.
- Begins to use the past tense of verbs: "Mommy closed the door," "Daddy went to work."
- Refers more frequently to the activities of others and to objects and events in the past.
- Changes tone of voice and sentence structure to adapt to listener's level of understanding: To baby brother, "Milk gone?" To mother, "Did the baby drink all of his milk?"
- Gives first and last name, sex, brothers' and sisters' names and telephone number.
- Answers appropriately when asked what to do if tired, cold or hungry.
- Recites and sings simple songs and rhymes.

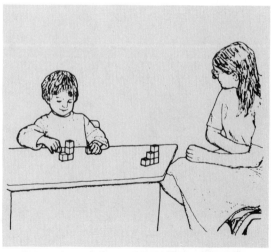

Answers questions about "how many"

Personal-Social Development

- Outgoing; friendly; overly enthusiastic at times.
- Moods change rapidly and unpredictably; laughing one minute, crying the next; may throw tantrum over minor frustrations (a block structure that will not balance); sulk over being left out.
- Imaginary playmates or companions are common; holds conversations and shares strong emotions with this invisible friend.
- Boasts, exaggerates and "bends" the truth with made up stories or claims of boldness.
- Cooperates with others; participates in group activities.
- Shows pride in accomplishments; seeks frequent adult approval.
- Often appears selfish; not always able to take turns or to understand taking turns under some conditions.
- Tattles on other children.
- Demands doing many things independently, but may have a near-tantrum when problems arise: paint that drips, paper airplane that will not fold right.
- Enjoys role-playing and make-believe activities.
- Relies (most of the time) on verbal rather than physical aggression; may yell angrily rather than hitting to make a point.
- Name-calling and taunting are ways of excluding children from friendship groups.
- Establishes close friendships with playmates; beginning to have a "best" friend.

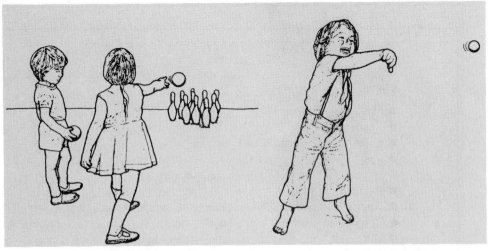

Cooperates with others   **Takes pride in accomplishments**

DAILY ROUTINES—FOUR-YEAR-OLDS

Eating

- Appetite fluctuates from very good to fair.
- May develop dislikes of certain foods and refuse them to the point of tears if pushed.
- Uses all eating utensils; becomes quite skilled at spreading jelly or peanut butter or cutting soft foods such as bread.
- Eating and talking get in each other's way; talking usually takes precedence over eating.
- Likes to help in the preparation of a meal: dumping premeasured ingredients, washing vegetables, setting the table.

Bathing Dressing, Toileting

- Takes care of own toileting needs; often demands privacy in the bathroom.
- Does an acceptable job of bathing and brushing teeth, but should receive some assistance (or subtle inspection) from adults on a regular basis.
- Dresses self without assistance; can lace shoes, button buttons, buckle belts. Gets frustrated if problems arise in getting dressed and may stubbornly refuse much-needed adult help.
- Can sort and fold own clean clothes, put clothes away, hang up towels, straighten room.

Sleeping

- Averages 10 to 12 hours of sleep at night; may still take an afternoon nap or quiet time.
- Bedtime usually not a problem if cues, rather than parents' orders, signal the command: when a particular TV show is over, when the story is finished, when the clock hands are in a certain position.
- Some children fear the dark but usually a light left on in the hall is all that is needed.
- Getting up to use the toilet at night may require helping the child settle down for sleep again.

Play and Social Activities

- Playmates are important; plays cooperatively most of the time; may be bossy.
- Takes turns; shares (most of the time); wants to be with children every waking moment.
- Needs (and seeks out) adult approval and attention; may comment, "Look what I did."
- Understands and needs limits (but not too constraining); will abide by rules most of the time.
- Brags about possessions; shows off; boasts about family members.

DEVELOPMENTAL ALERTS

Check with a health care provider or early childhood specialist if, by four years of age, the child *does not*:

- State own name in full.
- Recognize simple shapes: circle, square, triangle.
- Catch a large bounced ball.
- Speak so as to be understandable to strangers.
- Have good control of posture and movement.
- Hop on one foot.
- Appear interested in and responsive to surroundings.
- Respond to statements without constantly asking to have them repeated.
- Dress self with minimal adult assistance; manage buttons, zippers.
- Take care of own toileting needs; have good bowel and bladder control with infrequent accidents.

THE FIVE-YEAR-OLD

Five-year-old children are in a period of relative calm. There is greater emotional control. The child is friendly and outgoing much of the time, and is becoming remarkably self-confident and reliable. The world is expanding well beyond home and family and child-care center. Friendships and group activities are of major importance at this age.

Constant practice and mastery of skills in all areas of development is the major focus of the five-year-old. However, this quest for mastery coupled with a high energy level and robust self-confidence can lead to mishap. Their eagerness to do and explore often interferes with their ability to foresee danger or the potentially disastrous consequences of their own behavior. Therefore, the child's safety and the prevention of accidents must be a major concern of parents and caregivers. At the same time, adults' concerns must be handled in ways that do not interfere with the child's development.

DEVELOPMENTAL PROFILES AND GROWTH PATTERNS

Growth and Physical Characteristics

- Gains 4 to 5 pounds (1.8–2.3 kg) per year; weighs an average of 38 to 45 pounds (17.2–20.5 kg).
- Grows an average of 2 to 2.5 inches (5.0–6.4 cm) per year; is approximately 42 to 46 inches (106.7–116.8 cm) tall.
- Heart rate (pulse) is approximately 90–110 beats per minute.
- Respiratory rate ranges from 20–30 depending on activity and emotional status; pattern of breathing changes to thoracic (from the chest).
- Body temperature is stabilized at 98 to 99.4 F.
- Head size is approximately that of an adult's.
- May begin to lose "baby" (deciduous) teeth.
- Body is adult-like in proportion.
- Requires approximately 1700 calories daily.
- Visual acuity is 20/20 using the Snellen E chart.
- Visual tracking and binocular vision are well-developed.

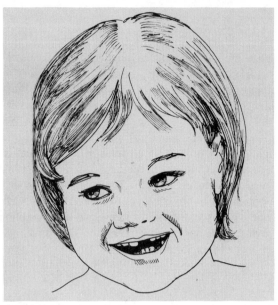

Begins to lose teeth

Motor Development

- Walks backwards, heel to toe.
- Walks unassisted up and down stairs, alternating feet.
- May learn to turn somersaults.
- Bends to touch toes without flexing knees.
- Walks a balance beam.
- Learns to skip using alternating feet.
- Catches a ball thrown from three feet away with accuracy.
- Rides a tricycle or wheeled toy with speed and skillful steering; some children learning to ride bicycles.
- Jumps or hops forward on both feet ten times in a row without falling.
- Balances on either foot with good control for ten seconds.
- Builds three dimensional structures with small cubes by copying from a picture or model.
- Reproduces many shapes and letters: square, triangle, *A, I, O, U, C, H, L, T, V, X, Y.*
- Demonstrates good control of pencil or marker; may begin to color within the lines.
- Cuts on the line with scissors (not perfectly).
- Hand dominance is definitely established.

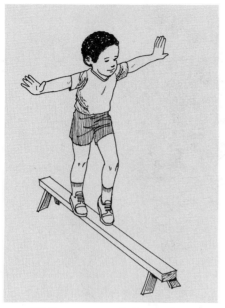

Walks across a balance beam

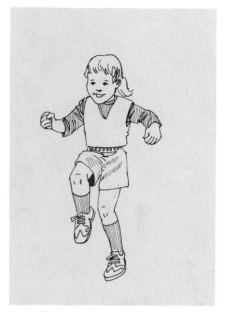

Balances on either foot

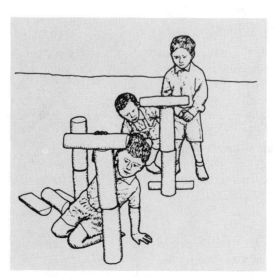

Builds structures from models

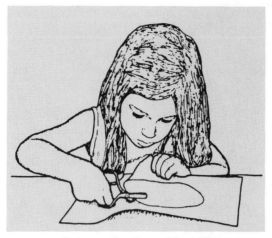

Cuts on the line with scissors

Perceptual and Cognitive Development

- Forms rectangle from two triangular cards.
- Builds steps with set of small blocks.
- Understands concept of same shape, same size.
- Sorts objects on the basis of both color and form.
- Sorts a variety of objects in such a way that all things in the group have a single common feature (classification skill: all are food items or boats or pieces of clothing).
- Does not yet recognize class inclusion; that is, when given a set of wooden beads with many red ones, a few blue ones, child can understand that all beads are wooden and some are red and some are blue, but when asked "Are there more red beads or more wooden beads?" the child replies, "More red ones."
- Understands the concepts of smallest and shortest; places objects in order from shortest to tallest, smallest to largest.
- Identifies objects with specified serial position: first, second, last.
- Rote counts to twenty and above.
- Recognizes numerals from one to ten.
- Understands the concept of less than, "Which bowl has less water?"
- Understands the terms dark, light, and early: "I got up early, before anyone else. It was still dark."
- Relates clock time to daily schedule: "It is time to turn on TV when the clock hands point to 5."
- Some children can tell time on the hour: five o'clock, two o'clock.
- Knows what a calendar is for.
- Recognizes and identifies penny, nickel and dime.
- Understands the concept of one-half; can say how many pieces an object has when its been cut in half.

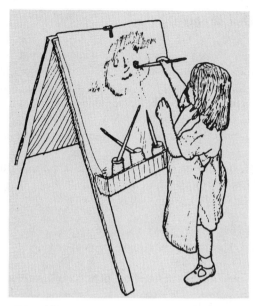

Identifies and names at least four colors

Speech and Language

- Vocabulary of 1500 words or more.
- Tells a familiar story using pictures.
- Defines simple words by function: A ball is to bounce; a bed is to sleep in.
- Identifies and names at least four colors.
- Recognizes the humor in simple jokes; makes up jokes and riddles.
- Produces sentences with an average length of 5 to 7 words.
- States the name of own city and town, birthday and parents' names.
- Answers telephone appropriately; calls person to phone or takes a brief message.
- Speech is nearly 100% intelligible.
- Uses "would" and "could" appropriately.
- Uses past irregular verbs consistently: "went," "caught," "swam," "gave."
- Uses past tense inflection (-ed) appropriately to mark regular verbs: "jumped," "rained," "washed."
- Understands the singular/plural contrast for nouns: *ball/balls, block/blocks, baby/babies.*

Personal-Social Development

- Enjoys friendships; often has one or two special playmates.
- Is often generous: shares toys, takes turns, plays cooperatively; has occasional lapses.
- Participates in group play and shared activities with the other children; suggests imaginative and elaborate play ideas.
- Is affectionate and caring, especially toward younger or injured children and animals.
- Generally does what parent or caregiver requests; follows directions and carries out responsibilities most of the time.
- Continues to need adult comfort and reassurance but may be less open in seeking and accepting comfort.
- Has better self-control; has fewer dramatic swings of emotions.
- Likes to tell jokes, entertain and make people laugh.
- Continues to ask many questions.
- Eager to learn new things, boastful about accomplishments.

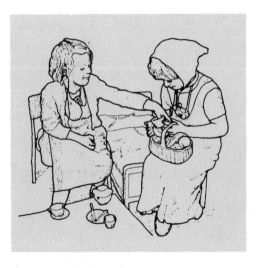

Participates in elaborate make-believe

DAILY ROUTINES—FIVE-YEAR-OLDS

Eating

- Eats well, but not at every meal.
- Likes familiar foods, prefers most vegetables raw.
- Latches on to food dislikes of family members and declares these as own dislikes.
- Makes breakfast (pours cereal, gets out milk and juice) and lunch (spreads peanut butter and jam on bread).

Sleeping

- Independently manages all routines associated with getting ready for bed; can help with younger brother or sister's bedtime routine.
- Averages 10 or 11 hours of sleep per night. The occasional 5-year-old still naps.
- Dreams and nightmares are commonplace with many children.
- Going to sleep is often delayed if the day had been especially exciting or exciting events are scheduled for the next day.

Bathing, Dressing, Toileting

- Takes full responsibility for own toileting; may put off going to the bathroom until an accident is barely avoided.
- Bathes fairly independently but needs some help getting started.
- Dresses self completely; learning to tie shoes, sometimes aware when clothing is on wrong side out or backwards.
- Careless with clothes; leaves them strewn about; needs many reminders to pick them up.
- Uses Kleenex, but often does a careless or incomplete job.

Play and Social Activities

- Helpful and cooperative in carrying out family chores and routines.
- Somewhat rigid about the "right" way to do something and the "right" answers to a question.
- Fearful that mother may not come back; very attached to home and family; willing to adventure to some degree but wants the adventure to begin and end at home.
- Plays well with other children, but three may be a crowd: two 5-year olds will often exclude the third.
- Shows affection and protection toward younger sister or brother, may feel overburdened at times if younger child demands too much attention.

DEVELOPMENTAL ALERTS

Check with a health care provider or early childhood specialist if, by five years of age, the child *does not*:

- Alternate feet when walking down stairs.
- Speak in a moderate voice; neither too loud, too soft, too high, too low nor monotone.
- Follow a series of 3 directions in order ("Stop, pick up the cup and bring it here").
- Use 4 to 5 words in acceptable sentence structure.
- Cut on a line with scissors.
- Sit still and listen to an entire short story (5 to 7 minutes).
- Maintain eye contact when spoken to (unless this is a cultural taboo).
- Play well with other children.
- Perform self-grooming skills independently—brush teeth, wash hands, comb hair.

REVIEW QUESTIONS

1. List three motor skills that appear between 2 and 5 years of age.
   a.

   b.

   c.

2. List a social/personal skill typical of each of the following ages.
   a. 3 year olds:

   b. 4 year olds:

   c. 5 year olds:

3. List three major speech and language skills in order of their appearance between 3 and 5 years of age.
   a.

   b.

   c.

TRUE OR FALSE

1. Growth is slow and even during most of the preschool years.

2. A full set of baby teeth is usually in place by 3 or 4 years of age.

3. Complete bladder control is achieved between 3 and 5 years of age.

4. 15 to 18 hours of sleep at night is characteristic of the older preschool age child.

5. Silly talk and silly jokes (that is, silly to adults) seem to go hand in hand with the development of language skills in the preschool age child.

6. Imaginary playmates are common among preschool age children.

7.   Fluctuations in appetite are perfectly normal during the preschool years.

8.   Safety and prevention of accidents need not concern adults because preschool-age children have learned to be cautious.

9.   It is most unusual for 5-year-olds to have dreams or nightmares.

10. Defining nouns by function (what the object does) is characteristic of the older preschool age child: "A kite is to fly," "A book is to read."

MULTIPLE CHOICE   Select one or more correct answers from the list below.

1.   Which of the following might be cause for concern if a three-year-old were *not* doing them?
     a.   talking clearly enough to be understood most of the time
     b.   stating own name
     c.   using scissors to cut out shapes accurately

2.   Which of the following might be of concern if a four-year-old were *not* doing them?
     a.   hopping on one foot
     b.   printing all letters of the alphabet legibly and in order
     c.   dressing self with only occasional help from the parent or caregiver

3.   Which of the fullowing might be cause for concern if a child were *not* doing them by age five?
     a.   listening to a story for 5 minutes
     b.   making an acceptable sentence using 4 or 5 words
     c.   alternating feet when walking down stairs

4.   Which of the following describe most healthy preschool age children?
     a.   eager to find out all about everything they contact
     b.   vocabulary and intellectual skills are expanding rapidly
     c.   content to stay close to adults; not willing to begin to branch out into activities with other children

5.   Which of the following expectations are unrealistic of preschool age children?
     a.   explaining why they did something unacceptable
     b.   being responsible for younger brothers and sisters
     c.   answering the telephone pleasantly

Chapter 6

An Overview: Six and Beyond

THE KINDERGARTEN–PRIMARY YEARS

The period following the preschool years is especially remarkable. All areas of development are working together smoothly. The child seems to be in a stage of developmental integration. Boys and girls alike can be depended upon to take care of their own personal needs—washing, dressing, toileting, eating, getting up and getting ready for bed. They carry out any number of family and school obligations. They observe family rules about mealtimes, television, and needs for privacy. They also run errands and carry out simple responsibilities at home and at school. In other words, these are children in control of themselves and their immediate world.

Above all, they are ready and eager to go to school, even though they become somewhat apprehensive when the time actually arrives. Going to school creates anxieties, such as getting to school on time, remembering to bring back assigned items, walking home alone or to after-school child care if that is a part of the daily routine. Throughout the early school years many children seem almost driven by the need to do everything right. On the other hand, they enjoy being challenged and completing tasks. They also like to make recognizable products and to join in organized activities. By and large, the early school years are an enjoyable experience for most children.

The end of the preschool years sees most of the large motor skills well-developed. The child can walk, run, jump, hop, kick and throw. All that is required is an abundance of practice through everyday experiences. It is largely through playful activities that children refine and elaborate basic skills. It is true that in some communities and school districts there is a push for early printing, reading and number work. However, most child developmentalists feel that children of five or six are not yet ready to take on the finer perceptual-motor tasks such as printing. (There are exceptions: children who ask to learn to print their own name or be shown how to write certain letters).

Letter and word reversals are one common example of perceptual-motor skills not yet fully developed. For the most part, such irregularities need not be worrisome; usually they correct themselves almost spontaneously. Within a short time, most children, if they have not been pressured, will matter-of-factly take on the writing tasks typical of primary classrooms. Others will reach this level of perceptual motor competence a bit later. With good teaching, most children, with few exceptions, do learn to print and write during the primary school years.

Most 6 and 7-year-old children are quite adept in other areas of perceptual development. They use their senses to extract all kinds of information from their environment.

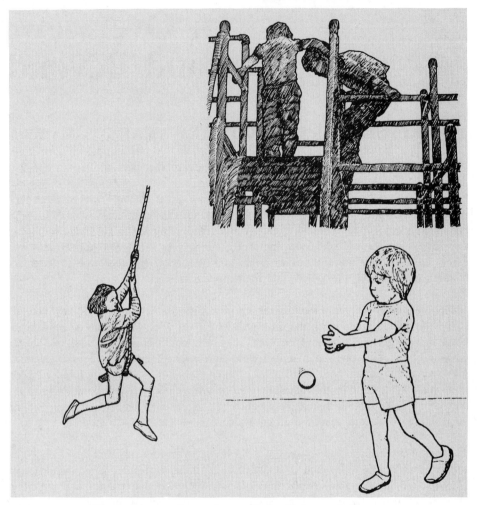

They can run, jump, hop, climb, kick, and throw.

These sensory activities are necessary if basic learning is to occur. Developmental kindergartens recognize such needs in young children. They emphasize and encourage children in the manipulation of all types of sensory materials—blocks, dramatic play, paints, puzzles, paste and paper, sand, water, cooking and science experiences.

Learning to read is the most complex perceptual task the child will encounter following the preschool years. It involves making fine discriminations among visual and auditory symbols—that is, learning to recognize the sight and sound of letters. It means, too, that children must learn to combine letters to form words. They must also learn to put these words together into intelligible thoughts that can be read or spoken. Yet, complex as the task is, most children between six and eight years of age become so adept at reading that it soon becomes a taken-for-granted skill.

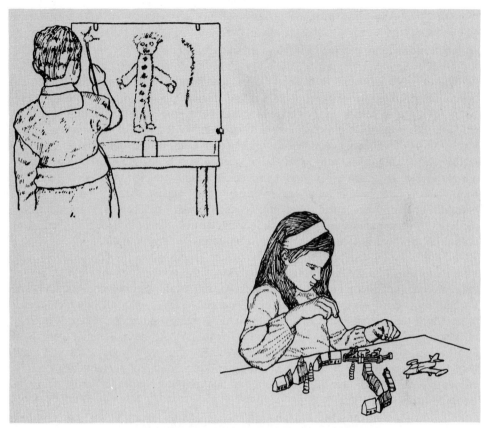

**Developmental kindergartens encourage
children in the manipulation of blocks,
dramatic play, and painting.**

Changes also are taking place in the way primary-age children think. They begin to realize that the values and viewpoints of others are often different from their own. In other words, children begin to place themselves in "another person's shoe." They also begin to use greater logic in their efforts to understand their world. Most children, for example, have become quite systematic in looking for a misplaced jacket or book. They no longer declare, as the preschooler so often does, that "someone stole it." Furthermore, there is some evidence of the following developing abilities:

- Planning ahead: "I'm going to save these books for when I stay with Grandmother";
- Understanding time and motion: "Cars go faster than bicycles";
- Remembering: "Can we go back to the zoo again?"
- Classifying: "All the mittens go in this box and all the caps in this one."

Primary age children love to flaunt their knowledge and will defend stubbornly what they think are facts. They will insist on the absolute "rightness" of each new bit of acquired information, especially if "teacher said so."

In spite of great individual differences, the language of 6- and 7-year-old children is much like that of adults. Furthermore, they are chatterboxes. They seem to talk incessantly, trying to dominate every conversation at home and school. It is this constant practice, however, that allows children to acquire an impressive vocabulary, learn various types of sentence construction, formulate all kinds of questions and be creative in the use of language. Many children between 6 and 8 continue to have perfectly normal speech irregularities, such as consonant substitutions: "Put the balentines in the vack room." Grammatical or syntactic irregularities appear often, especially over-generalizations of grammatical rules: "He broked the plate"; "The gooses swammed in the lake." With continuing experience these irregularities usually disappear of their own accord unless there is too much pressure from adults to "say it right."

Play continues to be the most important activity of the primary school child. It is the major avenue for fostering social development as well as all other developmental skills. For the most part, six-, seven- and eight-year-olds play well with other children, especially if the group is not too large and children are of similar age. There is a keen interest in making friends, being a friend, having friends. At the same time, there may also be a good deal of tattling, quarreling, bossiness and exclusiveness: "If you play with Linda then you're not *my* friend." Some children show considerable aggression. However, at this age it tends to be more verbal than physical, aimed at hurting feelings rather than doing physical hurt.

A major factor in forming friendships is proximity or availability. Friends are defined as someone who is "fun," "pretty," "strong" or someone who "acts nice." Friends are usually playmates that the child has ready access to in the neighborhood and at school. However, friendships at this age are easily established and readily abandoned, not stable or long-lasting.

Most children have had strong sex-role stereotypes stamped upon them long before the age of six. Even in today's world of greater equality between men and women, young children continue to make traditional role responses. They say that women will be teachers and nurses and men will be pilots and police officers; that boys are big, strong, loud and competent; that girls are small, quiet, obedient and cry a lot. Kindergarteners especially, seem to regard sex-role stereotypes as the absolute and only correct behavior. They may even try to enforce these stereotypes more rigidly than do adults: "Mommies *can't* be pilots." This suggests that it is perhaps a normal, even an essential, developmental process for young children to adopt rigid sex-role schemes for a time. These rigid schemes usually mellow as the child nears adolescence. Many of today's youth are highly androgynous; that is, young men and women alike can express both masculine and feminine traits by being compassionate and independent, gentle and assertive.

THE ELEMENTARY SCHOOL YEARS

Between eight and twelve years of age, friendships become more enduring. The child develops a truly mutual understanding and respect for the other person. Ways of thinking about themselves, others, and the world in general changes dramatically. During this period, the child learns more abstract ways of thinking, gains greater understanding about cause and effect, begins to use genuine logic in figuring out how things work. The child also comprehends that things really are the same in spite of being used for alternative purposes or seen from a different perspective—a shovel can be used not only for digging, but for prying; a soup bowl can be traced around to draw a circle.

The stretch of years from eight or nine to adolescence is usually enjoyable and peaceful for all concerned. The child has adjusted to being at school for six or more hours each day. The stresses, strains and frustrations of learning to read, write, do basic arithmetic and follow directions are long forgotten. Changes in physical growth and development are quite different from child to child during this period. Girls in particular grow more rapidly. According to recent research girls as young as 8 or 9 may already be experiencing some of the early hormonal changes associated with puberty.

And so, the era of childhood comes to an end. The first twelve years or so have been given over to dramatic changes. There has been the wondrous evolvement from a small, helpless infant into an adult-like individual capable of complex and highly coordinated motor, cognitive, language and social behaviors. As children approach adolescence and move through that stage of development before entering adulthood, there may again be frequent emotional upheavals, again be much questioning, searching and testing. Adolescents must discover once again, only at a different developmental level, who they are and how they fit into society. How well the adolescent weathers this developmental period depends on sound and healthy developmental experiences in the early years. That is why the focus of this handbook has been on portraying developmental patterns and sequences during the all-important first five years. It is these years that provide the foundation for healthy development throughout the entire life span.

REVIEW QUESTIONS

1. List three perceptual skills required in learning to read.
    a.

    b.

    c.

2. List three reasonable expectations for a 6 to 8 year old child in terms of home routines.
    a.

    b.

    c.

3. List three characteristics of being a friend and making friends among 6 to 8 year old children.
    a.

    b.

    c.

4. List three characteristics of the cognitive functioning of children between 8 and 12 years of age.
    a.

    b.

    c.

TRUE OR FALSE

1. During the early school years, most children are able to take care of their own personal needs—bathing, dressing, eating.

2. Play with blocks, sand and water, and housekeeping activities should be eliminated from kindergarten curriculum.

3. There is no evidence of logical thinking prior to the primary age years.

4. Sex-role stereotyping disappears completely by the time most children enter first grade.

5. Somewhere in the mid-elementary school years, children become quite skilled at looking at situations from another's point of view.

6. Between 9 and 12 years of age, many girls are beginning to show the results of early hormonal changes associated with puberty.

MULTIPLE CHOICE   Select one or more correct answers from the lists below.

1. During the primary years children can be expected to
   a. respect the privacy of others.
   b. take care of younger brothers or sisters in parents' absence.
   c. get themselves and younger brothers and sisters ready for school with no adult help or supervision.

2. Developmental kindergartens are characterized by
   a. giving direct instruction and drill in printing upper and lower case letters.
   b. providing reading instruction as soon as the child enters kindergarten.
   c. a belief that play should be an integral part of the kindergarten curriculum.

3. Six- seven- and eight-year-olds
   a. do a good bit of tattling and bossing.
   b. make friends easily and give them up just as easily.
   c. are seldom aggressive, either verbally or physically.

4. In terms of sex role stereotypes, kindergarteners
   a. may declare that "Mommies can't drive trucks" and "Daddies can't be nurses."
   b. are very rigid about sex-role stereotypes with anyone who attempts to reason with them.
   c. will never alter their sex-role concepts.

5. Grammatical irregularities during the primary years
   a. are not unusual.
   b. are a sign of abnormality; normally developing six- or seven-year-olds would never be heard to say, "The mouses falled into the water."
   c. should always be corrected and the child made to practice the correct form by repeating it at least ten times.

Chapter 7
When to Seek Help
for a Child

One of the most persistently asked questions is if a child is developing normally. It is a perplexing and difficult question, because of the range of normalcy and the great variation among children of the same general age. It is a question that requires thorough and on-going deliberation and investigation. At the same time, it is a question that must be answered quickly.

Developmental problems or delays, if they do exist, need to receive immediate attention. Research indicates that early identification and intervention can lessen the seriousness of a problem. Early intervention can also reduce, or prevent, negative impact on other areas of development. Reliable screening programs for children from birth through age five are widely available. Furthermore, federal legislation and money are available to assist in locating young children with developmental problems. The screening programs are often community sponsored or associated with public school systems.

Parents are usually the first to suspect a developmental problem or delay in their child. Those who do not are the exception. It is parents who become uneasy or fear that something is not quite right. Even so, they may not seek help immediately for a variety of reasons:

- Denial that the condition is anything to worry about
- Reluctance to openly acknowledge that a problem exists
- Uncertainty about how to locate professional help
- Uneasiness about seeking advice for a problem that is difficult to specifically identify or describe
- Self-doubt arising from having been told there is really no problem—that the child will eventually "outgrow" it
- Confusion over conflicting information given by clinicians
- Timidness about pressuring for further consultation.

Consequently, the problem often does not go away; instead, it worsens. For this reason parents must always be encouraged to talk about any misgivings or doubts they have about their child's development. Health-care professionals, teachers, caregivers—all who work or have contact with young children—must listen and be responsive to any concern parents express, directly or indirectly.

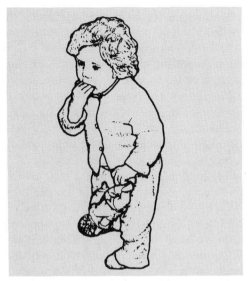

Signs of developmental problems may be subtle.

CAUSE FOR CONCERN

Deciding if a developmental delay or irregularity is of concern is not easy. True, some problems are so obvious they readily can be identified. The child with Down syndrome is easily recognized because of unique physical characteristics. However, the basis for determining many other developmental problems is not always so clear-cut. The signs may be so subtle, so hard to pinpoint, that it is difficult to clearly distinguish between children who definitely have a problem—the definite yes's—and those who definitely do not have a problem—the definite no's.

To determine if a delay or deviation is of real concern, several factors need to be considered:

- Children who exhibit signs of developmental problems in certain areas often continue to develop much like a normal child in other respects; such children present a confusing developmental profile.
- Great variation exists in the range of children's achievements within developmental areas; the rate of maturation is uneven and conditions in the child's environment are continually changing. Both maturation and environment interact to exert a strong influence on every aspect of the child's development.
- Developmental delays or problems may not be immediately apparent. Many children learn to compensate for slight deficiencies such as a mild to moderate vision or hearing loss. It is not until later, when the child is placed in structured and more demanding situations as in a first-grade reading class, that these deficiencies become obvious.

At what point should a hunch or uncomfortable feeling about a child's development be cause for concern and action? It seems safe to say that whenever a parent has feelings of uncertainty about a child's developmental progress or lack of progress, they should seek help. Parents who are uneasy about their child need to discuss their concerns with an early childhood specialist or health care provider. Together they can determine if developmental screening is warranted. Certainly, a developmental delay or irregularity demands investigation whenever it interferes with a child's ability to participate in everyday activities. In addition, the frequent occurrence or constant repetition of a troublesome behavior is often a reliable sign that help should be sought. Seldom, though, is a single incidence of a questionable behavior cause for concern. Of concern, too, is a child's continuing reluctance to attempt a new skill or to fully acquire a developmental skill. For example, a ten-month-old infant who tries to sit alone, but still must use hands for support may or may not have a problem. Clusters or groups of delays or developmental differences are always a warning sign, however. A ten-month-old infant who is not sitting without support, not smiling and babbling in response to others, almost surely is experiencing developmental difficulty. In either case, the need for developmental screening is indicated.

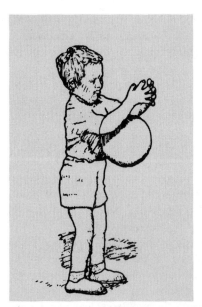

A child's reluctance to attempt new skills or to fully acquire a developmental skill is cause for concern.

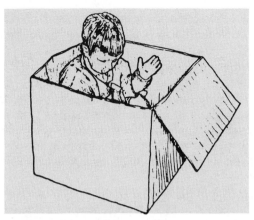

Noting and recording a child's behavior enables the evaluator to focus on what is actually occurring.

EVALUATING THE YOUNG CHILD

Several levels of information-gathering are involved in a comprehensive developmental evaluation. These include observation, screening, and diagnostic assessment. A combination of observation and screening techniques are useful for initial location and identification of individual children with possible delayed or abnormal development. Diagnostic assessment includes in-depth testing and careful interpretation of test results. Clinicians from various disciplines should participate in the diagnosis. It is their responsibility to provide detailed information about the problem areas and the specific nature of the child's problems. For example, a four-year-old child's delayed speech patterns may be noted during routine screening procedures. Subsequent diagnostic testing may pinpoint several other conditions: a moderate, bilateral hearing loss, (loss of hearing in both ears), a severe malocclusion (an overbite), withdrawn behaviors. Poor production of many letter sounds and an expressive vocabulary typical of a two-and-one-half-year-old may also be noted. These findings can then be translated into educational strategies and intervention procedures that will benefit the child's overall development.

The evaluation process always begins with careful and systematic observation. Noting and recording various aspects of a child's behavior enables the evaluator—parent, teacher, clinician—to focus on what is actually occurring. In other words, observations provide information about what the child can and cannot do. Observational data can be obtained by using simple checklists, frequency counts, or short written descriptions (anecdotal notes) of what a child does in a particular situation. Direct observation often confirms or rules out impressions or suspicions regarding a child's abilities. For example, a child may not count to five when asked to do so. That same child, however, may be observed to spontaneously and correctly count objects while at play. A child thought to be hyperactive may be observed to sit quietly for 5 to 10 minute stretches when given interesting and challenging activities, thereby ruling out hyperactivity.

Parents' observations are particularly valuable. They provide a kind of information and understanding that cannot be obtained from any other source. They also give insight into parents' attitudes, perceptions and expectations concerning the child. Involving parents in the observation phase of evaluation may help to reduce their anxiety. Even more important, direct observation often points up unrecognized strengths and abilities in a child. When parents actually see their child engaged in appropriate activities it may encourage them to focus more on the child's strengths and less exclusively on the child's shortcomings.

Screening procedures, together with careful observation, are an important first step in identifying developmental delays or problems. Screening tests assess a child's present level of performance. They evaluate the child's current abilities, deviations, delays and impairments in all major areas of development: fine and gross motor, perceptual-cognitive, speech and language, and personal-social adjustment. Information from a medical examination of the child, a health and developmental history (See Appendix 2 and Appendix 4) completed by the child's parent, a brief parent interview, and a vision and hearing evaluation present a fairly comprehensive picture of the child. If problem areas are identified during routine developmental screening, further diagnostic testing is indicated. It must be remembered, however, that *screening tests do not constitute a diagnosis*. Furthermore, screening tests should not be used as a basis for planning an intervention program. In every case, more than one instrument should be used to obtain

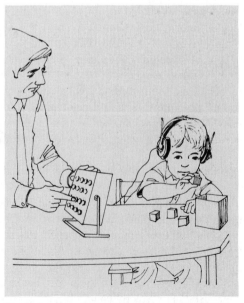

Participating in a pure-tone audiometric test

a clear and valid picture of the child's development. By using more than one type of test, the shortcomings or limitations inherent in any single screening instrument are reduced.

Screening Instruments

Several important criteria must be considered in selecting an appropriate screening instrument.

- Age of child
- Cultural background of the family
- Native language of the family and child
- Severity and nature of the child's developmental problem.

A number of comprehensive developmental screening instruments are available for use with young children; however, not all of them evaluate all developmental areas. Some instruments are criterion-referenced; that is, a child's performance is compared to certain predetermined standards. Criterion-referenced tests measure whether the child has mastered a given skill such as tying a bow, walking a balance beam, matching five shapes and colors. Other screening tests are norm-referenced. In norm-referenced tests the child's performance is compared to that of the "norm" or average performance of other children of the same age or sex: for example, the child can count a given number of pennies, identify letters of the alphabet, build a tower of 6 blocks.

A sample of screening instruments are listed below:

- Apgar Scale—a test to determine the physical status of the newborn. It evaluates muscle tone, respiration, color, heartbeat and reflexes at one and five minutes after birth.
- Neonatal Behavior Assessment Scale (Brazelton) with Kansas Supplements— provides a general assessment of overall behavioral responses to various stimuli in the full-term infant up to 28 days of age.
- Bayley Scales of Infant Development—useful for assessing all developmental areas in children birth through 2½ years.
- Brigance Diagnostic Inventory of Early Development—a criterion-based screening tool appropriate for assessing children 0–6 years; measures development in all major areas through observations of child's performance.
- Denver Developmental Screening Test (DDST)—a popular screening instrument that can be used with children 0–6 years to assess motor, language, cognitive and personal-social development.
- Developmental Profile 11—utilizes interviewing procedures to assess major developmental achievements in children 0–9 years.
- Peabody Picture Vocabulary Test (PPVT)—useful for evaluating the receptive and expressive vocabularies of children 2½–18 years.
- Learning Accomplishment Profile (LAP)—a screening tool for evaluating the developmental skills of handicapped and non-handicapped children 0–6 years.
- Home Observation for Measurement of the Environment (HOME)—an instru-

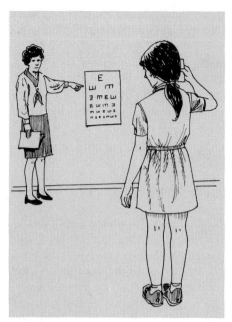

Vision screening is important for identifying problems.

ment for assessing the home environment and responsiveness of adult care providers to children 0–6 years.

- Uniform Performance Assessment System (UPAS)—a criterion-referenced tool that measures developmental skills of children 0–6 years in all major developmental areas.
- Denver Eye Screen Test (DEST)—an instrument for individualized vision screening of children six months and older.
- Snellen Illiterate E—a particularly useful vision-screening device for identifying vision acuity and potential muscle imbalance of the eyes in children 2½ and older.
- Pure Tone Audiometry—used to measure the responses of children 2½–18 years to a range of auditory tones; is especially useful for identifying children with middle ear problems.
- Sound localization—child turns to locate a source of sound: bell, voice, stereo speakers. While not a formal screening instrument, it is an effective method for screening hearing abilities of children 12 months to 2½ years.

Intelligence tests, such as the Wechsler Intelligence Scale for Children (WISC) and the Stanford-Binet Intelligence Scales, are sometimes given to young children. The purpose of IQ tests is to attempt to determine a child's ability to process information. The scores received on an IQ test are compared to scores of other children of the same age. These tests try to measure how much the child knows, how well the child solves

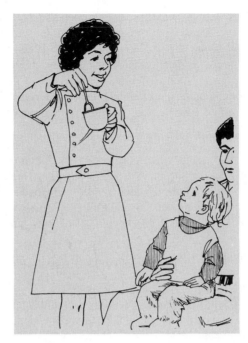

**Sound localization is useful for informal
testing of the young child's hearing.**

problems, and how quickly the child can perform a variety of cognitive tasks. IQ tests and the resulting scores must be used with caution, even skepticism, where young children are concerned.

The IQ scores of infants and preschool-age children *are not valid predictors* of future or even current intellectual performance. Even though intelligence is influenced to some unknown degree by heredity and maturation, measurement of intelligence is not a developmental issue; IQ tests do not measure the following:

- the opportunities the child has had to learn
- the quality of those learning experiences.

In general, standardized IQ tests do not account for these factors. Therefore, the use of a single IQ test score to determine a child's cognitive or intellectual skills *must always be challenged.*

Testing Results
The increasing and widespread use of developmental screening programs is of great benefit in detecting possible developmental problems in young children. However, the screening process itself can contribute to situations that may affect the outcome negatively. Children's attention spans are short and vary considerably from day to day, or

from task to task. Illness, fatigue, anxiety, lack of cooperation, irritability or restlessness can have a negative effect on performance. Unfamiliarity with the adult who is administering a test may prove to be a negative factor. Unfamiliarity with the test environment itself may result in poor performance. Young children frequently do not perform as well in a strange situation. Often they are capable of doing much better in a more comfortable situation. Consequently, *results derived from developmental screening assessments must be regarded with caution*. The following points are included to serve as reminders:

- Interpret and use test results with extreme caution. Avoid drawing hasty conclusions. Above all, do not formulate a diagnosis from limited information or a single test score. In analyzing screening results, recognize that developmental test results are strictly a measure of the child's abilities *at that given moment*. They may not be an accurate representation of the child's actual development or developmental potential. Only an *on-going* assessment can provide a complete picture of the child's developing skills and abilities.

- Recognize the dangers of labeling an individual child as learning disabled, mentally retarded or behavior disordered, especially on the basis of a single screening. Labels are of little benefit. They can and often do have a negative affect on both expectations for the child and ways that parents, caregivers and teachers respond to the child.

- *Question test scores*. Test results can be interpreted incorrectly. One test may suggest that a child has a developmental delay when actually there is nothing wrong. Such conclusions are called false-negatives. The opposite conclusion can also be reached. A child may have a problem that does not show up in the screening and so may be incorrectly identified as normal. This is a false-positive. The first situation leads to unnecessary anxiety and disappointment for the child's family, or even changes in the way they respond to their child. The latter situation—the false-positive—can lull a family into not seeking further help and so the child's problem worsens. Both of these situations could have been avoided with better testing and careful interpretation.

- Results from screening tests *do not* constitute a diagnosis. Additional information must be collected and in-depth clinical testing must be completed before a diagnosis is given or confirmed. Even then, errors may occur in diagnosing developmental problems. There are many reasons for misdiagnosis, such as inconsistent and rapid changes in a child's growth and developmental achievements or changing environmental factors, such as divorce.

- Failed items on a screening test do not dictate curriculum items or skills to be taught. The test skills are but single items representative of a broad range of skills to be expected in a given developmental area at an approximate age. A child who cannot stand on one foot for 5 seconds will not overcome a developmental problem by being taught to stand on one foot.

- And once again, test results do not predict the child's developmental future. As stressed earlier, screening tests measure a child's abilities and achievements at the time of testing. In many cases, the results do not correlate with subsequent testing. There is always the need for ongoing assessment and for in-depth clinical diagnosis when screening tests indicate potential problems and delays.

In the elementary grades, achievement tests are administered regularly by most school districts. These tests are designed to measure how much the child has been learning in school about specific subject areas. On such tests, the child is assigned a percentile ranking, based on a comparison with other children of the same grade level. For example, a child in the 50th percentile in math in doing as well as 50% of the children in the same grade.

CONCLUSIONS

Careful observation and developmental screening are integral parts of a comprehensive assessment of the young child. Such evaluations provide information about the status of the child, but only at the time of testing. Information obtained from observation and screenings, when used as an on-going process and interpreted judiciously, makes an important contribution to the overall assessment of a child's developmental status.

REVIEW QUESTIONS

1. List three ways that a parent may indicate anxiety about a possible developmental problem in their child.

   a.

   b.

   c.

2. List three reasons why one might expect a developmental problem in a young child.

   a.

   b.

   c.

3. List three ways for evaluating a child for a possible developmental disability.

   a.

   b.

   c.

4. List three major areas of development that can be assessed with the appropriate screening instrument.

   a.

   b.

   c.

5. List three infant screening instruments.

   a.

   b.

   c.

TRUE OR FALSE

1. Reliable screening programs for children, birth through 5, are not readily available.

2. It is always easy to tell the normally developing child from the child who is not developing normally.

3. Developmental problems always show up at birth or within the first few weeks of life.

4. Parents' observations of their child are of little value.

5. The Denver Developmental Screening Test (DDST) is used exclusively as a test of newborn abilities.

6. The results of IQ tests must always be viewed with caution and skepticism.

7. Effective diagnosis can be formulated on the basis of a single test score.

8. Screening tests measure a child's ability only at the time of testing.

9. Achievement test scores are often expressed in percentile ratings.

MULTIPLE CHOICE   Select one or more correct answers from the lists below.

1. Parents who fear something is wrong with their child
    a.   can be depended upon to seek help immediately.
    b.   may be uncertain about how to go about getting help.
    c.   may not seek further help because they have been told by a professional to stop worrying, that the child will "outgrow it."

2. It may be difficult even for professionals to identify developmental problems because
    a.   a child with a problem may be quite normal in many ways.
    b.   a child may have learned to compensate for a developmental problem (learned to work around it).
    c.   the child cannot talk and tell the professional what is wrong.

3. In evaluating the young child, first-hand observation is important because
    a. observation reveals what the child can actually do under everyday conditions.
    b. observations confirm or rule out suspicious or casual impressions about the child.
    c. a child may show skills during an observation session not exhibited during a formal testing situation.

4. Screening instruments include
    a. instruments designed to give a specific IQ score.
    b. instruments that measure only language performance.
    c. instruments designed to assess the home environment including aspects of parent-child interactions.

5. Infant screening tests
    a. are always predictive of a child's future performance as a teenager.
    b. measure both reflexive and voluntary motor behaviors.
    c. can and should be done within the first few minutes of life.

6. Test scores
    a. always provide accurate assessment of the child's abilities and should never be questioned by parents or caregivers.
    b. often reflect how the child is feeling on a given day, rather than his or her best performance.
    c. are sufficient for formulating a complete diagnosis and treatment guide for children with developmental problems.

Chapter 8

Where to Go for Help

Referral and treatment are required when screening tests, assessments or other evaluations point to the possibility of a developmental problem in a young child. Without immediate follow-up and intervention services, parents often feel helpless, confused and anxious. They may even feel guilty about their child's problem. Children, in turn, may become equally confused and anxious because they sense subtle (or not so subtle) changes in their parents' expectations and attitudes toward them.

THE DEVELOPMENTAL TEAM

Effective treatment of a developmental problem or delay requires the pooling of knowledge. There must be collaboration among practitioners and agencies that specialize in serving young children and their families. A child's growth and development depends upon a balanced interrelatedness of the various developmental areas. A delay in one area invariably interferes with development in other areas, just as progress in one supports progress in others. If a three-year-old has a hearing loss, the child is likely to have problems with language, as well as with cognitive and social development. The ability to hear well is central to language development and language development is central to both cognitive and social development. The services of an audiologist, speech and language therapist, psychologist, early childhood teacher and, perhaps, a social-service agency, may all be required to provide adequate intervention services for this three-year-old hearing-impaired child. Communication and cooperation among specialists and agencies providing services to young children is essential if the team approach is to benefit the child's overall development. Information must be shared, services coordinated and duplication avoided.

Parent involvement in the assessment and intervention procedures cannot be omitted. Parents have valuable information to contribute. In addition, many parents are able to learn and apply various therapy recommendations at home. Sustained interest and participation in their child's intervention program is achieved if the developmental team abides by the following:

- Keeps parents informed;
- Explains rationales for treatment procedures;
- Points out and emphasizes the child's progress;
- Teaches the parents ways of working with their child at home (if the parent is able to do so);
- Provides parents with positive feedback for their continued efforts on behalf of the child.

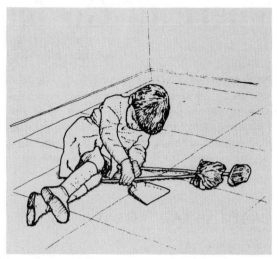

Identifying the problem: This child has cerebral palsy.

REFERRALS

The referral process first involves identifying the problem. The second step is to put parents and child in touch with educational programs and appropriate clinical services. Clinicians who need to see the child may include a pediatrician, dentist, ophthamologist, perceptual-motor specialist, speech therapist and dietician.

Initially, the child's strengths, weaknesses and developmental needs are evaluated by the assessment team. The next step is to carefully match the child to services and educational programs available in the community. The family's financial resources and ability to provide transportation must also be taken into consideration. If a family cannot afford special services, has no knowledge of financial assistance programs and does not own a car, it is unlikely that the family can carry out recommendations for treatment. Rarely are such problems insurmountable, however. Most communities have social-service agencies that can help families find and make use of needed services.

After an intervention program has been planned, a team coordinator, often called a case manager, works with the family. The case manager helps the family to establish initial contacts and set up arrangements with the recommended services and agencies. At this point, many parents may become overwhelmed. They find the task of approaching multiple agencies and surmounting bureaucratic red tape more than they can manage. Many do not or cannot complete the arrangements unless they receive additional help. Therefore, a follow-up telephone call from the case manager is important. The call can remind and motivate parents to make final arrangements. Assistance can be given to parents with problems they may already have encountered. The need for a case manager

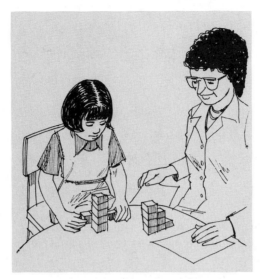

The classroom teacher and other members of the developmental team assume responsibility for conducting periodic reviews of the child's progress.

is so crucial that it has been written into recent federal legislation (PL 99-457) designed to help families and young children with developmental problems.

Placing the child in an early childhood educational setting is a frequent recommendation of a developmental team. In that setting, the classroom teacher and other members of the developmental team assume responsibility for conducting periodic reviews of the child's progress. The appropriateness of current placements and special services are evaluated on an on-going basis. In this way it can be determined whether the child's needs are being met. Throughout, there must be continuing communication and encouragement between teachers, practioners and parents. Parents' understanding of the values of a program or special service are improved if one or both parents are contacted regularly. Frequent contacts also reinforce parents' cooperation and help to ensure that the intervention program is of maximum benefit to the child.

RESOURCES

Many kinds of resources are available to families, caregivers, and teachers who work with children with (or at-risk for) developmental problems. These resources are provided at the local, state and national levels. They fall into two major categories: those that provide direct services and those that provide information.

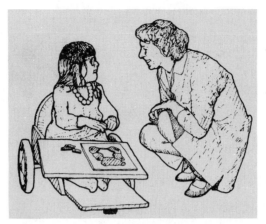

Services for children with developmental problems are available from a variety of agencies.

Direct Services

Numerous agencies and organizations provide direct services and technical assistance. They help not only young children with developmental problems but also their families and early childhood educators and caregivers working with such children. In addition, these agencies are a valuable referral source. Generally, they are aware of existing networks of services, agencies and qualified specialists. A sample of agencies and individuals who provide direct services to children follows:

- Public health departments at city, county or state levels;
- Local public school systems, especially the special services division;
- Hospitals and medical centers;
- Well-child clinics;
- University affiliated services (UAF's);
- Head Start programs;
- Mental health centers;
- Child Find screening programs;
- Early childhood centers and schools for exceptional children;
- Practioners from many disciplines: pediatricians, nurses, psychologists, audiologists, ophthamologists, educators, early-childhood specialists, speech and language therapists, occupational and physical therapists, social workers.

Local service groups are also an important resource. Many of these organizations provide specific types of services. These include financial assistance, transportation, location of necessary resources, and the purchase of special equipment.

A number of national organizations provide direct assistance to children and families with specific needs:

- Parents of Down Syndrome Children;
- American Foundation for the Blind;
- Association for Children with Learning Disabilities;
- United Cerebral Palsy Foundation;
- National Society for Autistic Children;
- International Parents Organization (Deaf);
- Epilepsy Foundation of America;
- National Easter Seal Society for Crippled Children.

Their current addresses can be found at the local public library.

In addition, there are programs and agencies whose purpose is to give direct, technical assistance to educational programs and agencies serving young children with developmental problems. Many of these organizations also provide a variety of instructional materials. A sample of such agencies includes the following:

- National Information Center for Handicapped Children and Youth (NICHCY);
- Head Start Resource Access Projects (RAPs). Their purpose is to help Head Start programs provide comprehensive services to children with developmental problems;
- National Early Childhood-Technical Assistance System (NEC-TAS). This agency provides many kinds of assistance to federally funded handicapped children's projects;
- American Printing House for the Blind. This group produces a variety of materials and services for children with visual impairments. Materials include talking books, magazines in braille, large-type books and other materials such as a textbook, *The Visually Impaired Child, Growth, Learning, Development: Infancy to School Age*, intended for educators of blind and visually impaired children.

A variety of support services and organizations are also available in most communities. These are designed to help families cope with the special challenges and demands of caring for a child with developmental problems. The stress level among these families is often great. A child's developmental problems have impact on every member of the family and cause inescapable adjustments in family lifestyles. However, many emotional and financial problems can be eased or avoided altogether if the family is given early assistance and support. Assistance can take the form of marriage counseling, financial management, respite care, mental-health counselling, medical care, or help with transportation, household chores, laundry and child care.

Support groups are another service-oriented resource. They provide opportunities for parents to share their experiences with families having similar problems and concerns. Parents can be supported as they work toward strengthening their parenting skills. They can also be helped to learn and practice more effective ways to manage and discipline their child with special needs.

Information

Outstanding information from a variety of disciplines is published for parents, caregivers, and professionals who work with children with developmental problems. Professional journals, government publications, and reference books are available in most public libraries. These can be readily located with the help of a librarian. Special interest groups and professional organizations also provide a wealth of printed materials focused on high-risk children and children with developmental delays. Only a few are listed here:

- Professional journals and periodicals, such as the *Journal of the Division for Early Childhood, Topics in Early Childhood Special Education, Exceptional Children,* and *Teaching Exceptional Children;*
- Trade magazines for parents such as *Parents of Exceptional Children* and *Parents Magazine;*
- Government documents, reports and pamphlets. These are available on almost any topic related to child development, child care, early intervention, parenting, and every type of developmental problem. Publications can be purchased through the Superintendent of Documents, U.S. Government Printing Office, Washington, D.C., 20402; many are available in local government buildings;
- Bibliographic indexes and abstracts usually located in university, college and large public libraries. These are particularly useful to students and practioners who need to locate quickly what is available on a specific topic. Two of many examples are the following:
  - *The Review of Child Development*
  - *Current Topics in Early Childhood Education*
- Information searches and retrievals are available to locate data-based information collected from many sources including journals, books, government documents, commercial materials, and newsletters. Two examples are:
  - *ERIC* (Education Resources Information Center)—A major clearinghouse for information related to children. Its findings are published in the catalogue, *Clearinghouse on Elementary and Early Childhood Education;*
  - CEC Information Services (Council for Exceptional Children)—provides bibliographies related to prevention and early identification of developmental problems. One such reference is the *Exceptional Children Education Resources* (ECER).

National associations that focus entirely or in part on children with developmental problems are yet another resource. They often provide printed materials and sponsor annual conferences for students, educators, practioners, parents and caregivers. Such organizations include the following:

- Council for Exceptional Children (CEC), especially the Division for Early Childhood (DEC) within the Council;
- National Association for the Education of Young Children (NAEYC);
- National Association for Retarded Citizens (NARC);

- American Association on Mental Deficiency (AAMD);
- Children's Defense Fund.
- American Speech, Language and Hearing Association
- National Society for Autistic Children.

LEGISLATION

Several pieces of landmark legislation have been enacted on behalf of infants and young children over the past twenty years. The resulting policies and programs are intended to lessen the extent and permanency of developmental problems through prevention and through early identification and intervention. Significant legislative acts include the following:

- P.L. 88-452 (1965): This law was passed as a section of the antipoverty reform of the 1960's. Parts of this law provided for the establishment of Head Start programs. It also included provisions for developmental screening, comprehensive medical and dental services, nutritious meals, and compensatory early education for young children living near or below the poverty level. In 1972 and 1974 the act was amended so that handicapped children would also be served.
- The National Program for Early and Periodic Screening, Diagnosis and Treatment (EPSDT) (1967): This program is designed to evaluate children at developmental risk from a physical and psychological perspective, and also to address the needs of the family.
- Supplemental Feeding Program for Women, Infants and Children (WIC) (1972): This law created a medically prescribed nutrition program designed to improve maternal health during pregnancy, to promote full-term prenatal development and to increase birth weight of newborns. It is also aimed at improving the general health of infants and young children who receive inadequate nutrition, which puts them at risk for developmental problems.
- PL 94-142 (1975): The Education for All Handicapped Children Act includes special preschool incentive monies. The intent of this legislation is to motivate states to locate and provide comprehensive treatment and educational services for young children with or at-risk for developmental problems.
- PL 99-457 (1986): Essentially this is an amendment to PL 94-142. This law makes special and emphatic provisions related to young children with developmental problems or at high-risk for such problems. Individualized Family Service Plans (IFSP) are an integral part of the mandated services. The IFSP is to be written by an interdisciplinary team and services are to be coordinated by a case manager. All states receiving federal money under PL 99-457 must establish programs for eligible 3 to 5 year old children by the 1990–1991 school year. If they fail to do so, their early childhood handicapped funding will be terminated. The law also provides funds for states who wish to provide services to infants (0 to 3 years) who are at-risk for or already exhibiting developmental problems.

CONCLUSIONS

In conclusion, finding help for children with developmental problems is not a simple matter. The issue is complex; some children present tangles of interrelated developmental problems. These problems seem to multiply during the crucial first five years of a child's life if not dealt with as early as possible. Effective intervention must be comprehensive, integrated, and on-going. In addition, it must be directed toward not just one or two developmental areas, but to all areas at the same time. This requires team work on the part of specialists from many disciplines, agencies and organizations working cooperatively with the child and family. It also requires that everyone involved with the child be aware of the available resources and know how to tie in with them. Everyone involved must have a working knowledge of the legislative acts that help to provide services for children with developmental problems and their families.

REVIEW QUESTIONS

1. List three of the several professions that routinely serve on a developmental team.
   a.

   b.

   c.

2. List three responsibilities of a developmental team.
   a.

   b.

   c.

3. List three sources of direct, hands-on services for a child and family with developmental problems.
   a.

   b.

   c.

4. List three organizations that focus solely on specific handicapping or disabling conditions.
   a.

   b.

   c.

5. List three pieces of federal legislation enacted since 1970 that serve young children who are at-risk for or have a handicapping condition.
   a.

   b.

   c.

TRUE OR FALSE

1. Parents never feel guilty about their child's problems, especially when they could not possibly have caused it.

2. A delay or problem in one developmental area almost always affects other developmental areas.

3. Because of high costs, there is no clinical help available for a disabled child if a parent is out of work or living at the poverty level.

4. Case managers are an unnecessary expenditure, even a luxury, on a developmental team.

5. There are few government documents or publications suitable for use by parents, caregivers or teachers.

6. WIC is a piece of federal legislation aimed at helping unskilled mothers learn a self-supporting job skill.

7. Effective intervention must be concerned with all areas of development simultaneously.

8. Child Find programs are aimed at locating missing children.

9. Placement in early childhood educational programs is a frequent recommendation of a developmental child-study team.

10. Parents have no role in screening or intervention procedures until the professionals have completed their work-up and inform parents of the results.

MULTIPLE CHOICE   Select one or more correct answers from the lists below.

1. If a young child has an undetected hearing loss that child is likely to have additional problems with
   a. language development.
   b. social development.
   c. cognitive development.

2. The following organizations provide assistance to disabled children and their families
   a. National Society for Autistic Children
   b. Audobon Society
   c. Epilepsy Foundation of America

3. The role of the case manager is to
   a. assist parents through the team process.
   b. keep parents informed of each step the team takes on behalf of the child.
   c. reprimand parents when they fail to keep records or appointments with the team members.

4. The referral process includes
   a. identification of a child's problem.
   b. decisions as to which professionals should see the child.
   c. helping find transportation for those families who cannot find it for themselves.

5. P.L. 99-457, enacted in 1986, mandates
   a. an individual service plan for the family as a whole.
   b. federal money for setting up early identification and intervention programs within each state.
   c. stiff fines (even imprisonment) for parents or teachers who do not report a disabling condition to the proper authorities.

Summary of Reflexes

Age	Appears	Disappears
birth	swallow*, gag*, cough*, yawn*, blink* suck rooting startle Moro grasp stepping plantar elimination Tonic neck reflex (TNR)	
1–4 months	Landau tear* (cries with tears)	grasp suck (becomes voluntary) step root Tonic neck reflex (TNR)
4–8 months	parachute palmar grasp pincer grasp	Moro
8–12 months		palmar grasp plantar reflex
12–18 months		
18–24 months		Landau
3–4 years		parachute elimination (becomes voluntary)

*Permanent; present throughout person's lifetime.

Developmental Checklists

A simple checklist, one for each child, is a useful observation tool for anyone working with infants and young children. The questions on the checklists that follow can be answered in the course of a child's everyday activities over a period or a week or more. "No" answers signal that a problem may exist and further investigation is probably a good idea. Several "no" answers indicate that additional investigation is a necessity.

The "sometimes" category is also an important one. It suggests what the child can do, at least part of the time, or under some circumstances. The "sometimes" category provides space where brief notes and comments can be recorded about how and when a behavior occurs. What the child may need is more practice, incentive, or adult encouragement. Hunches often provide a good starting point for working with the child. Again if "sometimes" is checked a number of times, further investigation is in order.

The observation checklists may be duplicated and used as part of the assessment process. A completed checklist contains information about a child that members of a developmental team would find useful in evaluating a child's developmental status and in determining an intervention program.

Child's Name _____ Age _____

Observer _____ Date _____

DEVELOPMENTAL CHECKLIST

BY 12 MONTHS: Does the Child	Yes	No	Sometimes
Walk with assistance?			
Roll a ball in imitation of an adult?			
Pick objects up with thumb and forefinger?			
Transfer objects from one hand to other hand?			
Pick up dropped toys?			
Look directly at adult's face?			
Imitate gestures: peek-a-boo, bye-bye, pat-a-cake?			
Find object hidden under a cup?			
Feed self crackers (munching, not sucking on them)?			
Hold cup with two hands; drink with assistance?			
Smile spontaneously?			
Pay attention to own name?			
Respond to "no"?			
Respond differentially to strangers and familiar persons?			
Respond differentially to sounds: vacuum, phone, door?			
Look at person who speaks to him or her?			
Respond to simple directions accompanied by gestures?			
Make several consonant-vowel combination sounds?			
Vocalize back to person who has talked to him or her?			
Use intonation patterns that sound like scolding, asking, exclaiming?			
Say "da-da" or "ma-ma"?			

Child's Name _____ Age _____

Observer _____ Date _____

DEVELOPMENTAL CHECKLIST

BY TWO YEARS: Does the Child Walk alone?	Yes	No	Sometimes
Bend over and pick up toy without falling over?			
Seat self in child-size chair? Walk up and down stairs with assistance?			
Place several rings on a stick?			
Place 5 pegs in a peg board?			
Turn pages 2 or 3 at a time?			
Scribble?			
Follow one-step direction involving something familiar: "Give me—." "Show me—." "Get a—."			
Match familiar objects?			
Use spoon with some spilling?			
Drink from cup holding it with one hand, unassisted?			
Chew food?			
Take off coat, shoe, sock?			
Zip and unzip large zipper?			
Recognize self in mirror or picture?			
Refer to self by name?			
Imitate adult behaviors in play— for example, feeds "baby"?			
Help put things away?			
Respond to specific words by showing what was named: toy, pet, family member?			
Ask for desired items by name: (cookie)?			
Answer with name of object when asked "What's that"?			
Make some two word statements: "Daddy bye-bye"?			

Child's Name _____ Age _____

Observer _____ Date _____

DEVELOPMENTAL CHECKLIST

BY THREE YEARS: Does the Child	Yes	No	Sometimes
Run well in a forward direction?			
Jump in place, two feet together?			
Walk on tiptoe?			
Throw ball (but without direction or aim)? Kick ball forward?			
String 4 large beads?			
Turn pages in book singly?			
Hold crayon: imitate circular, vertical, horizontal strokes?			
Match shapes?			
Demonstrate number concepts of one and two? (Can select one or two; can tell if one or two objects.)			
Use spoon without spilling?			
Drink from a straw?			
Put on and take off coat?			
Wash and dry hands with some assistance?			
Watch other children; play near them; sometimes join in their play?			
Defend own possessions?			
Use symbols in play—for example, tin pan on head becomes helmet and crate becomes a space ship.			
Respond to "Put—in the box," "Take the—out of the box"?			
Select correct item on request: big vs little; one vs two?			
Identify objects by their use: show own shoe when asked, "What do you wear on your feet"?			
Ask questions?			
Tell about something with functional phrases that carry meaning: "Daddy go airplane." "Me hungry now"?			

Child's Name _____ Age _____

Observer _____ Date _____

DEVELOPMENTAL CHECKLIST

BY FOUR YEARS: Does the Child	Yes	No	Sometimes
Walk on a line?			
Balance on one foot briefly? Hop on one foot?			
Jump over an object 6 inches high and land on both feet together?			
Throw ball with direction?			
Copy circles and crosses?			
Match 6 colors?			
Count to 5?			
Pour well from pitcher? Spread butter, jam with knife?			
Button, unbutton large buttons?			
Know own sex, age, last name?			
Use toilet independently and reliably?			
Wash and dry hands unassisted?			
Listen to stories for at least 5 minutes?			
Draw head of person and at least one other body part?			
Play with other children?			
Share, take turns (with some assistance)?			
Engage in dramatic and pretend play?			
Respond appropriately to "Put it beside," "Put it under"?			
Responds to two step directions: "Give me the sweater and put the shoe on the floor"?			
Respond by selecting the correct object—for example, hard vs. soft object?			
Answer "if," "what," and "when" questions?			
Answer questions about function: "What are books for"?			

DEVELOPMENTAL CHECKLIST

BY FIVE YEARS: Does the Child	Yes	No	Sometimes
Walk backward, heel to toe?			
Walk up and down stairs, alternating feet?			
Cut on line?			
Print some letters?			
Point to and name 3 shapes?			
Group common related objects: shoe, sock and foot; apple, orange and plum?			
Demonstrate number concepts to 4 or 5?			
Cut food with a knife: celery, sandwich?			
Lace shoes?			
Read from story picture book—in other words, tell story by looking at pictures?			
Draw a person with 3 to 6 body parts?			
Play and interact with other children; engage in dramatic play that is close to reality?			
Build complex structures with blocks or other building materials?			
Respond to simple three step directions: "Give me the pencil, put the book on the table, and hold the comb in your hand"?			
Respond correctly when asked to show penny, nickle, and dime?			
Ask "How" questions?			
Respond verbally to "Hi" and "How are you"?			
Tell about event using past and future tense?			
Use conjunctions to string words and phrases together—for example, "I saw a bear and a zebra and a giraffe at the zoo"?			

Child's Name _____ Age _____

Observer _____ Date _____

DEVELOPMENTAL CHECKLIST

BY SIX YEARS: Does the Child	Yes	No	Sometimes
Walk across a balance beam?			
Skip with alternating feet?			
Hop for several seconds on one foot?			
Cut out simple shapes?			
Copy own first name?			
Show well-established handedness; demonstrate consistent right or left handedness?			
Sort objects on one or more dimensions: color, shape or function?			
Name most letters and numerals?			
Count by rote to 10; know what number comes next?			
Dress self completely; tie bows?			
Brush teeth unassisted?			
Have some concept of clock time in relation to daily schedule?			
Cross street safely?			
Draw a person with head, trunk, legs, arms and features; often add clothing details?			
Play simple board games?			
Engage in cooperative play with other children, involving group decisions, role assignments, rule observance?			
Use construction toys, such as Leggos, blocks, to make recognizable structures?			
Do 15 piece puzzles?			
Use all grammatical structures: pronouns, plurals, verb tenses, conjunctions?			
Use complex sentences: carry on conversations?			

Growth Charts
For Boys And Girls

LENGTH BY AGE PERCENTILES FOR GIRLS AGED BIRTH-36 MONTHS

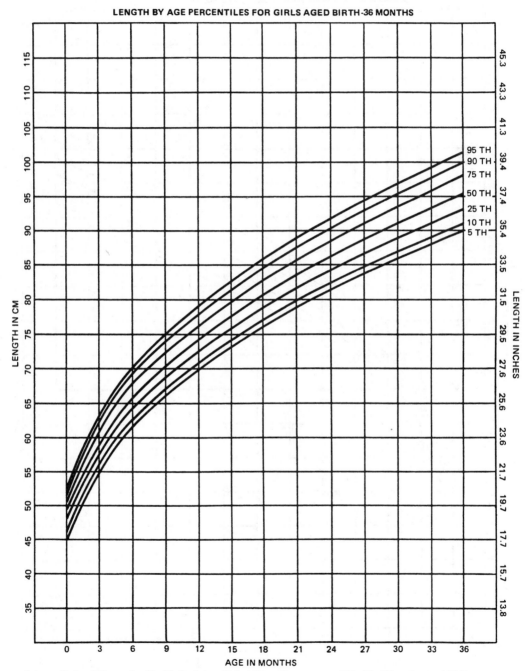

Source: National Center for Health Statistics, United States Department of Health, Education, and Welfare.

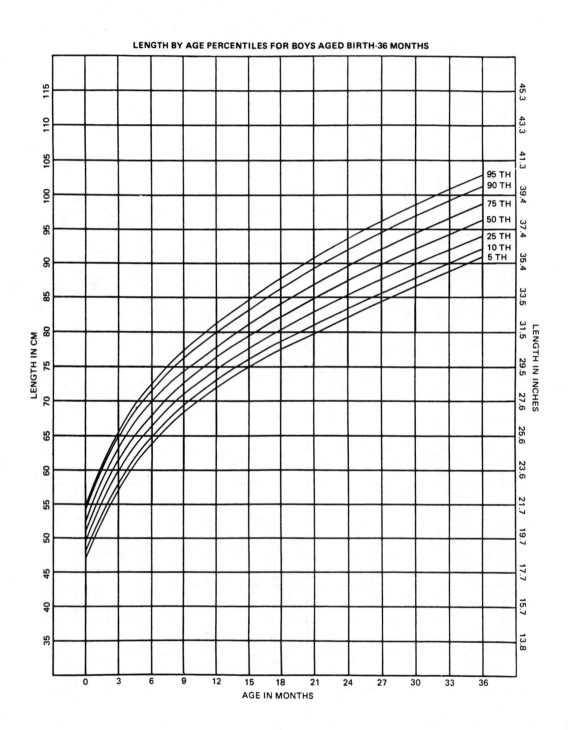

LENGTH BY AGE PERCENTILES FOR BOYS AGED BIRTH-36 MONTHS

WEIGHT BY AGE PERCENTILES FOR GIRLS AGED BIRTH-36 MONTHS

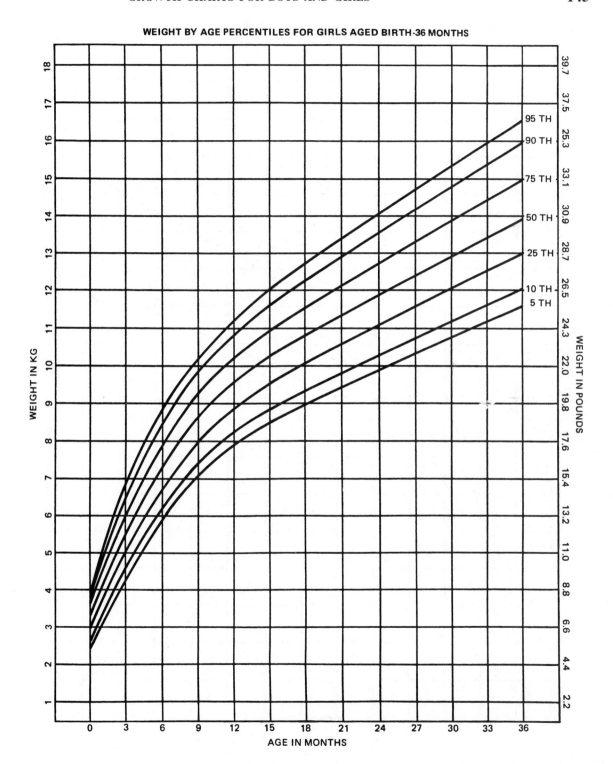

WEIGHT BY AGE PERCENTILES FOR BOYS AGED BIRTH-36 MONTHS

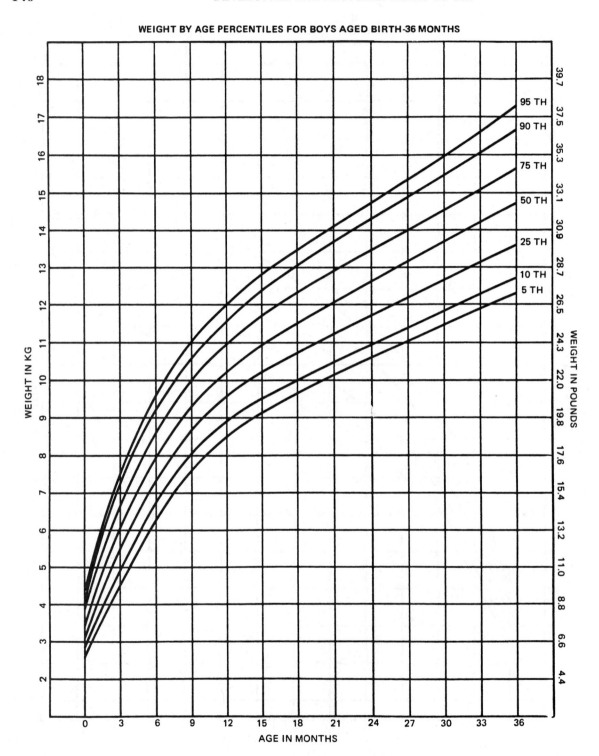

WEIGHT BY AGE PERCENTILES FOR GIRLS AGED 2 TO 18 YEARS

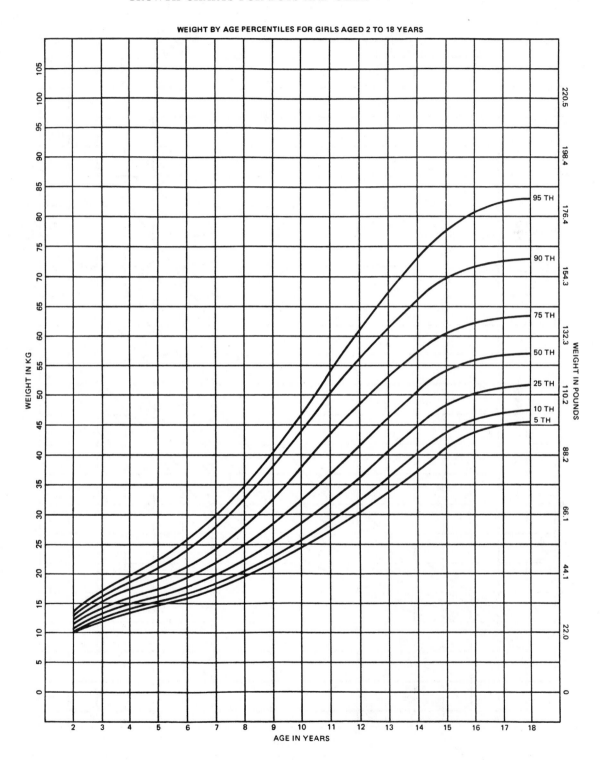

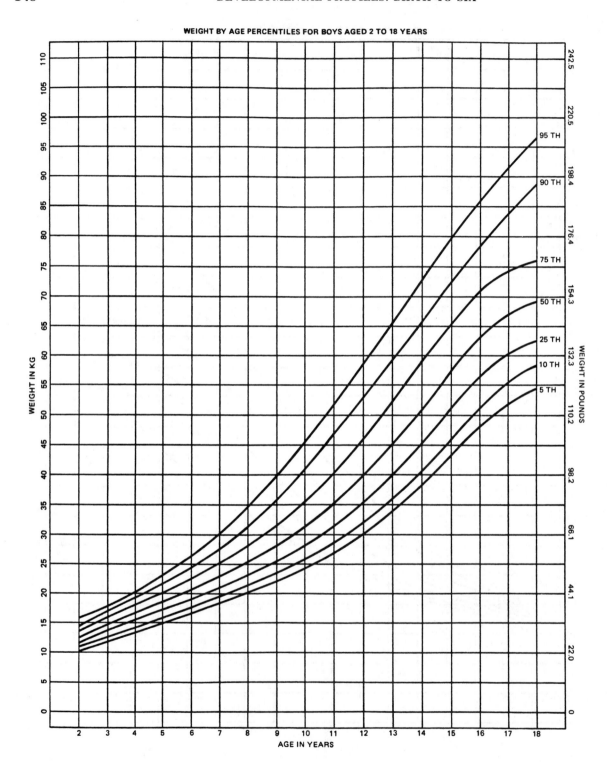

WEIGHT BY AGE PERCENTILES FOR BOYS AGED 2 TO 18 YEARS

STATURE BY AGE PERCENTILES FOR GIRLS AGED 2 TO 18 YEARS

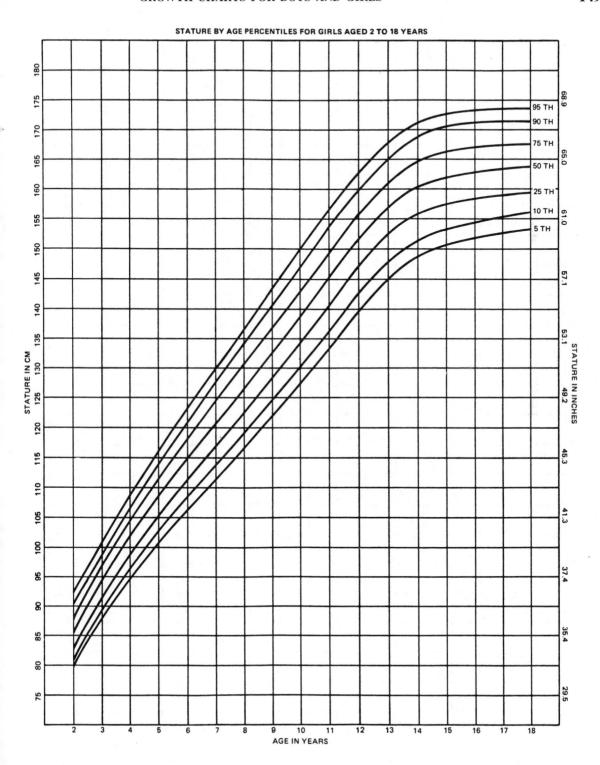

STATURE BY AGE PERCENTILES FOR BOYS AGED 2 TO 18 YEARS

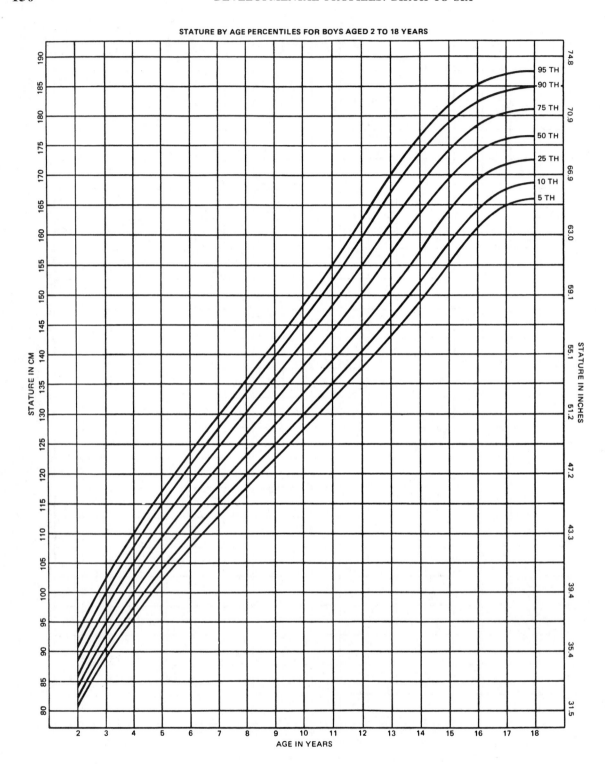

Child Health History

We appreciate your taking time to fill out this form as completely as possible. The information will be treated in a confidential manner and used for evaluating and for planning your child's program.

GENERAL INFORMATION

1. Child's Name _____ , _____ .
   (First)   (Last)

2. Child's Address _____ .
   (Street)

   _____ .
   (City, State, Zip)

3. Home Telephone Number (___) _____ .

4. Child's Sex: _____ Female _____ Male

5. Child's Date of Birth _____ _____ _____
   Month   Date   Year

6. Mother's Name _____ .

7. Father's Name _____ .

BIRTH HISTORY

8. Length of Pregnancy: ____ 6 ____ 7 ____ 8 ____ 9 months

9. Child's weight at birth: ____ lbs. ____ ozs. or ____ kilograms

10. _____ yes _____ no Were there any unusual factors or complications during

    this pregnancy? Please describe.

    _____ .

11. Did your child have any medical problems at the time of birth—for example, jaundice, difficulty breathing, birth defects? Please describe: _____

_____ .

12. What doctor is most familiar with your child? _____ .

Doctor's telephone number: _____ .

13. Does your child take any medication on a regular basis? ___ yes ___ no If yes,

name of medication and dosage: _____ .

14. Has your child had any of the following illnesses (dates)?

_____	measles	_____	rheumatic fever
_____	mumps	_____	chicken pox
_____	whooping cough	_____	pneumonia
_____	middle ear infection (otitis media)	_____	hepatitis
_____	meningitis		

15. Were there any complications with these illnesses, such as high fever, convulsions, muscle weakness, and so on. Please describe: _____ .

16. _____ yes _____ no Has your child ever been hospitalized? _____ Number of

times _____ Total length of time.

Reasons: _____ .

17. ___ yes ___ no Has your child had any other serious illness or injuries that

did not involve hospitalization?

18. How many colds has your child had during the past year?

19. Does your child have:

___ yes ___ no Allergies? To: (please specify)

Foods _____

Animals _____

Medicine _____

_____ yes _____ no Asthma?

_____ yes _____ no Hayfever?

20. _____ yes _____ no Has your child had any problems with earaches or ear

infections? If YES, how often in the past year? _____ .

21. _____ yes _____ no Has your child's hearing been tested?

When _____ _____ Was there any evidence of
          (month)   (year)

hearing loss (describe)? _____ .

22. _____ yes _____ no Does your child currently have tubes in his or her ears?

23. Do you have any concerns about your child's speech or language development?

_____ yes _____ no If YES, describe: _____ .

24. _____ yes _____ no Has your child's vision been tested?

Date of test: _____ month _____ year

25. _____ yes _____ no Was there any evidence of vision loss?

Please describe: _____ .

26. Does your child do some things that you find troublesome?

Please describe: _____ .

27. Has your child ever participated in out-of-the-home child care services—for

example, sitter, day care, preschool? Describe: _____ .

CHILD'S PLAY ACTIVITIES

28.   Where does your child usually play—for example, backyard, kitchen, bedroom?

   _____ .

29.   Does your child usually play: _____ alone? _____ with 1–2 other

   children? _____ with brothers/sisters?

   _____with older children? _____ with younger children?

   _____ with children of the same age?

30.   Is   your   child   usually   _____   cooperative?   _____   shy?

   _____ aggressive?

31.   What are some of your child's favorite toys and activities?

   Please describe: _____ .

32.   Are there any particular behaviors you would like us to watch?

   Describe: _____ .

CHILD'S DAILY ROUTINE

33.   Do you have any concerns about your child's:

   _____ eating habits?

   _____ sleeping habits?

   _____ toilet training?

   If YES, please describe: _____ .

34.   _____ yes _____ no Is your child toilet trained. If YES, how often does

   your child have an accident? _____ .

35.   What word(s) does your child use or understand for: urination _____

   bowel movement _____ .

36. How many hours does your child sleep? At night _____ ?

Goes to bed at: _____ p.m. Awakens at: _____ a.m.

Afternoon nap: _____ .

37. When your child is upset, how do you comfort him or her?

_____ .

38. The term "family" has many different meanings. Since the topic of families and family members is often included in classroom discussions, please list or describe who your child considers to be "family" at home. _____

_____

39. How many brothers and (or) sisters does your child have?
Brothers: (ages)   Sisters: (ages)

_____   _____

_____   _____

_____   _____

40. What language(s) is/(are) most commonly spoken in your home?

English _____ Other _____ .

Annotated Bibliography

CHILD DEVELOPMENT

Bee, H. *The developing child—fourth edition.* New York: Harper and Row Publishers, Inc., 1985.

This is an excellent text written by a sensitive child developmentalist who is a master at combining theory and research into readily understood application to the lives of everyday children and their parents.

Bower, T.G.R. *The perceptual world of the child.* Cambridge, MA: Harvard University Press, 1977.

Readable texts on perceptual development are most difficult to find but the Bower text, even though more than a decade old, is excellent—highly readable and still current in its coverage of the major aspects of perceptual development.

Charlesworth, R. *Understanding child development.* Albany, NY: Delmar Publishers, Inc., 1987.

An excellent book for teachers, caregivers and parents that focuses on growth and development of the infant, toddler and preschool child. A wealth of basic information is combined skillfully with numerous suggestions for working with young children.

Crain, W. C. *Theories of development.* Englewood Cliffs, NJ: Prentice Hall, 1980.

For those in need of a comprehensive introduction to major developmental theories, this text is exceptionally thorough and useful.

The Diagram Group. *Child's body.* New York: Paddington Press, 1977.

Not a new book, but especially useful to parents and caregivers in that it is filled with practical information about physical development, health and nutrition.

Flavell, J.H. *Cognitive development.* Englewood Cliffs, NJ: Prentice Hall 1985.

No text on cognitive development escapes being somewhat technical but this one, written by one of the leading researchers in cognitive/developmental theory is one of the least difficult because of its easy, anecdotal style.

Rice, M.L. and Kemper, S. *Child language and cognition.* Austin, TX: Pro-Ed, 1984.

This clearly written text assesses the relationship between children's linguistic and cognitive abilities in the early stages of language acquisition and discusses issues in both normal and atypical language development (graduate or professional level student).

Santrock, J.W. *Children.* Dubuque, IA: Wm. C. Brown Publishers, 1988.

A contemporary textbook that addresses current issues in child development and incorporates some of the latest research findings as well as traditional theories.

White, B.L. *The first three years of life.* Englewood Cliffs, NJ: Prentice Hall, 1977.

Though published a number of years ago, this is still a wonderfully practical book that describes the first three years of life and includes many useful recommendations about toys, games and activities, including those that are available commercially.

CHILDREN WITH DEVELOPMENTAL PROBLEMS OR AT HIGH-RISK FOR DEVELOPMENTAL PROBLEMS (IDENTIFICATION AND INTERVENTION)

Adler, S. and King, D., eds. *A Multidisciplinary treatment program for the preschool exceptional child.* Springfield, IL: Charles C. Thomas, 1986.

This text is a comprehensive, interdisciplinary manual on the care, education and treatment of young children with developmental problems; directed to professionals, day care providers and parents.

Allen, K.E. *Mainstreaming in early childhood education.* Albany, NY: Delmar Publishers, Inc, 1980.

This text provides a comprehensive overview of early intervention and early childhood education for children with developmental problems, as well as their inclusion in the integrated (mainstreamed) classroom. (Currently in revision).

Blackman, J.A. *Medical aspects of developmental disabilities in children birth to three.* Rockville, MD: Aspen Systems Corp., 1984.

This is an outstanding book for early childhood personnel as it provides well-illustrated and readily understood information about medical issues that affect the developmental progress of young children; highly recommended.

Fallen, N.F. & Umansky, W. *Young children with special needs.* Columbus, OH: Charles E. Merrill, 1985.

This text is especially useful for its focus on the developmentally different child as being in need of a "holistic" approach to early care and education just as is the normally developing child.

Hanson, M.J. and Harris, S.R. *Teaching the young child with motor delays.* Austin, TX: Pro-Ed, 1986.

This easy-to-read handbook bridges the gap between parents and professionals who work with motor-impaired children, birth to three, and includes teaching strategies and therapy activities to be used in the home and in the infant center.

Haslam, R.H.A. and Valletutti, P.J. *Medical problems in the classroom.* Austin, TX: Pro-Ed, 1985.

This book provides teachers and professionals from other disciplines with clues to early identification and points out ways that teachers can assist in the management of these problems.

Krajicek, M.J. and Tomlinson, A.I.T. *Detection of developmental problems in children.* Baltimore, MD: University Park Press, 1983.

Practical and readable, this is a highly acclaimed pediatric nursing text that focuses on early identification, screening and beginning intervention stategies with children with potential or identified developmental problems.

McCormick, L. and Schiefelbusch, R.L. *Early language intervention.* Columbus, OH: Charles E. Merrill, 1984.

A good introduction to both normal and atypical language development and overall communication development with practical examples of programs, procedures and materials for fostering communication skills in young children.

Peterson, N.L. *Early intervention for handicapped and at-risk children*. Denver, CO: Love Publishing Company, 1987.

This is an excellent text for students and professionals in early childhood special education and related disciplines who are working with young children with developmental problems; gives an invaluable perspective on what early intervention actually entails.

INFANTS, TODDLERS AND PARENTS

Apgar, V. and Beck, J. *Is my baby all right? A guide to birth defects*. New York: Trident, 1972.

This continues to be one of the best sources for information about genetic and environmental causes of developmental problems and what the progress and treatment of a problem is from birth on; sensitive and readable.

Brazelton, T.B. *Infants and mothers: Differences in development*. New York: Dell, 1969.

Though this book was published a number of years ago it remains one of the best descriptions of the first year of life. It is written by a sensitive and observant pediatrician who has remained at the forefront of developmental pediatrics.

Brazelton, T.B. *Toddlers and Parents*. New York: Dell, 1974.

Like Brazelton's infant book this is an exceptionally good book for parents and caregivers of young children; just as sensitively written as the earlier book, this one too, is a treasury of good advice and sensible suggestions about toddlers.

Bricker, D.D. *Early education of at-risk and handicapped infants, toddlers, and pre-school children*. Glenview, IL: Scott, Foresman, and Company, 1986.

Written by one of the leading infant specialists, this text offers both students and practitioners a contemporary view of the field with examples of application for those working with atypical infants and children.

Bromwich, R.M. *Working with parents and infants*. Austin, TX: Pro-Ed, 1981.

This remains one of the best books in the field for helping parents learn to work with their handicapped or high-risk children; particularly noteworthy is the inclusion of case histories covering successful, partly successful, and unsuccessful interventions; invaluable for those working with parents.

Caplan, F. and Caplan, T. *The first twelve months of life* and *The second twelve months of life*. New York: Putnam Publishing Co., 1982.

Very readable books that provide excellent descriptions of normal growth and development although their emphasis on month to month changes rather than on developmental sequence may contribute to some undue anxiety in new parents. Includes many practical suggestions for dealing with daily behaviors and routines.

Hanson, M.J. *Atypical infant development*. Austin, TX: Pro-Ed, 1984.

This interdisciplinary text presents students and professionals with a current review of research and literature on both normal and atypical infant development and suggests models and practices for application to programs for infants with developmental problems.

Leach, P. *Your baby and child from birth to age five*. New York: Alfred A. Knopf, 1986.

This book offers parents and caregivers excellent developmental explanations as well as practical suggestions for daily caregiving routines, appropriate play equipment and behavior management.

Marotz, L.; Rush, J. and Cross, M. *Health, safety and nutrition for the young child*. Albany, NY: Delmar Publishers, Inc., 1989.

This book provides a comprehensive overview of the factors that contribute to maximizing the growth and development of each child. It includes some of the most current research information and knowledge concerning each of these areas and is especially useful for teachers, caregivers and parents.

Wilson, L.C. *Infants and toddlers*. Albany, NY: Delmar Publishers, Inc., 1986.

Parents and caregivers will find this book particularly useful in understanding developmental sequences, creating enriching environments and providing appropriate learning experiences for infants and toddlers based on their developmental needs.

INDEX

161